RECHARGE
the
POWER
NAP

Kevin B DiBacco

Copyright © 2024 by Kevin B. DiBacco

All right reserved
ISBN: 9781964482491

TRIBUNE PUBLISHER

DISCLAIMER

No part of this publication may be reproduced in any form or by any means, including printing, scanning, photocopying, or otherwise, without the prior written permission of the copyright holder. The author has tried to present information that is as correct and concrete as possible. The author is not a medical doctor and does not write in any medical capacity. All medical decisions should be made under the guidance and care of your primary physician. The author will not be held liable for any injury or loss that is incurred to the reader through the application of the information here contained in this book. The author points out that the medical field is fast evolving with newer studies being done continuously, therefore the information in this book is only a researched collaboration of accurate information at the time of writing. With the ever-changing nature of the subjects included, the author hopes that the reader will be able to appreciate the content that has been covered in this book. While all attempts have been made to verify each piece of information provided in this publication, the author assumes no responsibility for any error, omission, or contrary interpretation of the subject present in this book. Please note that any help or advice given hereof is not a substitution for licensed medical advice. The reader accepts responsibility in the use of any information and takes advice given in this book at their own risk. If the reader is under medication supervision or has had complications with health-related risks, consult your primary care physician as soon as possible before taking any advice given in this book.

"The information and advice contained in this book are based upon the research and the personal and professional experiences of the author. They are not intended as a substitute for consulting with a healthcare professional. The publisher and author are not responsible for any adverse effects or consequences resulting from the use of any of the suggestions, preparations, or procedures discussed in this book. All matters pertaining to your physical health should be supervised by a healthcare professional."

ABOUT THE AUTHOR

Chapter 1. The Timeless Allure of the Midday Nap

Chapter 2. The Science Behind Napping

Chapter 3. Naps overall effect on the body

Chapter 4. The Power of Napping for Healing

Chapter 5. Historical Perspective on Napping

Chapter 6. Napping Techniques and Strategies

Chapter 7. Why is napping such a powerful tool?

Chapter 8. Napping for Creative Problem-Solving

Chapter 9. Napping as a catalyst for innovation

Chapter 10. Napping for Energy Restoration

Chapter 11. Napping as a sustainable energy source

Chapter 12. Implementing Strategic Napping:

Chapter 13. The Role of Napping in Regulating
Cortisol Levels

Chapter 14. Light Napping of 20–30 Minutes Ideal

Chapter 15. Napping Techniques:

Chapter 16. How napping improves memory consolidation

Chapter 17. The Healing Power of Naps:

Chapter 18. Napping's impact on cardiovascular health

Chapter 19. Napping as a Lifestyle Choice

Chapter 20. Advocating for napping rights in the workplace

Chapter 21. Napping habits for different age groups

Chapter 22. Napping etiquette in public spaces

Chapter 23. The Future of Napping

Chapter 24: Embracing the Nap Revolution: A Brighter Future for Well-being

ABOUT THE AUTHOR

Kevin understands adversity and the temptation to quit better than most. His life has been a testament to the power of perseverance despite severe hardship. Now, he shares his story and tools to inspire others to get off the mat when knocked down by life.

Kevin's health struggles began early, needing major surgery at just 16 years old. In his 20s and 30s, he endured 6 knee operations, 2 back surgeries, including spinal fusion, 2 hip replacements, and treatment for an aggressive brain tumor. Enduring over 10 major medical procedures would be enough to make anyone want to give up. Even as he was writing this, Kevin was struck by Covid-19. As if that wasn't another setback, Kevin developed Pneumonia and spent the spring of 2022 and the summer of 2023 having to get daily nebulizer treatments. Once again, his theories were put to the test. Once again, they worked!

But Kevin refused to see himself as a victim of circumstance. Through each diagnosis and rehabilitation, he consciously worked to reframe adversity as an opportunity for growth. Instead of sadly ruminating on limitations, he focused positively on each small win: standing, walking, and climbing stairs: during recovery. He visualized himself healed and happy against all odds.

Kevin leaned on his deep faith and the support of loved ones during the darkest times. When fear or hopelessness crept in, he prayed for the strength to take the next step forward. He turned to uplifting books and sayings for encouragement. Slowly but surely, he reclaimed his active lifestyle step by step.

Through his journey, Kevin realized firsthand the power of mindset to figure out one's life experience. He discovered that he could transform his outer reality by controlling his inner world: his thoughts, beliefs, and visualizations. Now, he hopes to share these lessons with others facing major life challenges.

Kevin's book recounts his medical battles, along with the techniques he used to stay grounded in positivity. He provides exercises to overcome negative self-talk, face fears, and visualize desired outcomes. Kevin believes we can all learn to reframe difficulties as growth opportunities. Wherever we feel like quitting, he urges us to proclaim, "I will keep going!"

Kevin's dramatic story provides living proof that, regardless of what knocks us down, we can choose to get back up. We all have access to inner reserves of strength to endure the unendurable. Kevin hopes his book will inspire others to fight major life battles to find their power to keep progressing. By committing to personal growth, we can overcome any obstacle, including those within our minds.

Chapter 1. The Timeless Allure of the Midday Nap

For millennia, cultures across the globe have cherished the restorative power of the afternoon siesta. This time-honored ritual of stealing a brief respite in the middle of the day dates to the ancient Egyptians, who sought refuge from the sweltering heat on cool stone pillows as early as 1500 BC. The Greeks and Romans also heartily embraced the nap, with luminaries like Aristotle and Plato extolling the virtues of a post-lunch slumber. Beds and couches were even expressly designed for languid lounging.

As civilization marched forward, the nap stayed a steadfast companion. Pious monks napped according to strict schedules in the Middle Ages, while wealthy nobles followed suit, indulging in sumptuous feasts and lengthy siestas. From the sun-dappled streets of Spain to the rolling hills

of Italy to the bustling markets of China, the nap was woven into the very fabric of daily life.
In Spain, the sobremesa reigns supreme, a languorous affair stretching from 2-4pm. Italians treasure their riposo as a hallmark of civility and key to proper digestion. Greek workers have even enshrined the right to nap in their employment contracts! Across Latin America, entire families retreat home for comida and 2–3-hour siesta. And in China and Japan, a quick post-lunch snooze is seen as essential nourishment for the mind and soul.

Alas, the nap fell out of favor in 20th century America, a casualty of the relentless march of office culture. Stigmatized as a mark of indolence, incompatible with the Puritan work ethic, the poor nap was banished. But like a persistent dream, it would not be denied. Science soon came to the nap's defense, with studies proving its potent ability to sharpen focus and boost productivity. Slowly but surely, progressive companies began embracing the power nap, carving out cozy spaces for weary workers.

And so, the nap endures, an ancient rite that speaks to our primal need for rest and renewal. In a world that never stops spinning, the midday nap is still a timeless oasis, a chance to pause, reset, and appear refreshed, ready to face whatever the afternoon may bring. A nap is not a relic of the past, but a gift for the ages, as essential to our well-being as the very air we breathe.

Chapter 2. The Science Behind Napping

Napping has been a part of human culture for centuries, and the benefits of a good nap are well-documented. But what exactly happens in our bodies and minds when we take a nap? In this subchapter, we will explore the science behind napping and shed light on how it can have a profound impact on our productivity and well-being.

When we sleep, our brain goes through various stages, including REM (rapid eye movement) and non-REM sleep. Napping, depending on its duration, can help us enter these stages and experience their unique benefits. For instance, a short power nap of 10–20 minutes can enhance alertness and improve motor skills. This is because it primarily involves non-REM sleep, which helps in memory consolidation and rejuvenation of the mind.

The Science Behind Napping

On the other hand, longer naps of 60–90 minutes (about 1 and a half hours) can include REM sleep, which is associated with dreaming and emotional processing. These naps can enhance creativity, problem-solving abilities, and boost overall mood. The inclusion of both REM and non-REM sleep in longer naps allows for a more comprehensive recovery of the body and mind.

Furthermore, napping can also positively affect our physical health. It has been shown to reduce the risk of heart disease, lower blood pressure, and improve immune system function. This is because during sleep, our body repairs and regenerates cells, resulting in improved overall health and well-being.

Napping also plays a crucial role in combating sleep deprivation, a prevalent issue Today. By taking a nap, we can compensate for lost sleep and recharge our energy levels. This, in turn, can lead to increased focus, enhanced cognitive abilities, and improved memory retention.

The Science Behind Napping

The benefits of napping are backed by extensive research. Scientists have used tools like EEGs, fMRIs, and PET scans to understand what is happening in the brain during nap periods. These studies have shed light on the unique brain wave patterns and changes in neurochemistry that underlie the restorative powers of napping.

For example, researchers at the University of California, Berkeley found that napping can improve the brain's ability to integrate new information and enhance memory processes. Their studies using electroencephalography (EEG) proved that naps as short as 10 minutes could induce brain wave patterns key for solidifying memories and integrating knowledge.

Other neuroimaging studies have revealed how napping can reduce levels of specific neurotransmitters linked to stress, while boosting neurotransmitters involved in memory consolidation. The changes in these brain chemicals may explain the stressbusting and brain-boosting benefits of napping.

The Science Behind Napping

Genetic research has also provided insights into the biological bases of napping. Scientists have found several genes related to sleep and circadian rhythms that may influence individual differences in best nap durations and responses. This emerging field sheds light on why some people get greater cognitive boosts from brief power naps, while others benefit more from longer naps.

Understanding these biological mechanisms helps confirm why napping feels restorative and clarifies the science behind harnessing naps for improved well-being. The research makes clear that napping is not a sign of laziness, but rather a way of optimizing brain function, enhancing alertness, joining memories, and regulating stress.

While more research is still needed, the existing science gives us a window into the measurable physical and neurological effects that enable napping to elevate our productivity and wellness. The field of napping neuroscience continues to evolve as researchers use modern technologies and genetic insights.

But the takeaway is clear: napping is far more than just sleep. It is a precise tool to recalibrate our minds, support cognitive functioning, aid memory and learning, energize the body, and regulate emotion. Understanding science empowers us to strategically use naps to enhance our health, productivity, and happiness, as well as support the well-being of our communities.

The science behind napping reveals measurable benefits for bodies, brains, and lives. Research continues to affirm napping's remarkable power to restore mental clarity, solidify memories, improve learning, enhance creativity, uplift mood, boost immunity and reduce stress. By understanding the biological mechanisms at play, we can improve napping and harness this practice that has been part of human history for millennia. Science is our guide to using naps as a precise tool for enhancing productivity, health, and wellness in the modern world.

The Science Behind Napping

Understanding the Sleep Cycle

To fully grasp the POWER of a NAP, it is crucial to understand the intricacies of the sleep cycle. Sleep is an essential part of our daily routine, allowing our bodies and minds to rest, repair, and rejuvenate. But what exactly happens during this seemingly passive state? Let's delve into the fascinating world of the sleep cycle.

The sleep cycle consists of several distinct stages that repeat throughout the night, each with its purpose and characteristics. The first stage is known as the non-rapid eye movement (NREM) stage. During this first phase, our brain activity slows down, and we gradually enter a relaxed state. This is the time when our body repairs itself, and our immune system strengthens.

As we progress into the deeper stages of NREM sleep, our brain waves become slower, and our breathing and heart rate decrease. It is during this period that our body releases growth hormones, promoting physical development and repair. Moreover, our brain merges memories and processes information, enhancing our cognitive abilities.

After approximately 90 minutes (about 1 and a half hours), we enter the rapid eye movement (REM) stage of sleep, which is characterized by increased brain activity and vivid dreaming. This stage is crucial for our emotional well-being, as it helps regulate our emotions and process experiences from the day. REM sleep also plays a vital role in learning and creativity, as it aids in problem-solving and critical thinking.

The sleep cycle is not linear; it repeats several times throughout the night. In the early cycles, we spend more time in deep NREM sleep, while REM sleep becomes more prominent in later cycles. This is why it is essential to have enough uninterrupted sleep, as it allows us to complete multiple sleep cycles and reap the maximum benefits of each stage.

Understanding the sleep cycle is the key to harnessing the POWER of a NAP. By strategically timing our naps, we can tap into the restorative effects of the sleep cycle, even during the daytime. Short power naps can help us recharge and improve our alertness, memory, and overall cognitive function. However, it is important to avoid long naps, as they can disrupt our regular sleep patterns and leave us feeling groggy.

Scientists have used innovative tools like electroencephalography (EEG) to study the sleep cycle and its distinct brain wave patterns. During NREM sleep, EEG readings show slower theta and delta brain waves, showing deep relaxation. In REM sleep, EEG shows increased beta wave activity like wakefulness, linked to heightened cognition and dreaming.

Understanding how sleep stages correspond to neural oscillations seen on EEG allows researchers to map the sleep cycle's impact on brain function. It also sheds light on how naps may refine brain performance. A NASA study found that a 26-minute nap improved pilots' alertness by 54% and performance by 34%, with EEG showing boosted brain activity.

The Science Behind Napping

Advances in neuroimaging have further illuminated how our sleeping brain runs. Studies using functional MRI show deactivated regions during NREM sleep associated with focus, problem-solving and handling emotions. This helps explain why deep sleep combines learning. REM sleep shows increased activation in visual areas, supporting complex dream imagery.

The discovery of sleep regulating chemicals like adenosine and melatonin has also advanced our grasp of sleep cycles. Adenosine builds up during waking hours, inducing drowsiness and regulating sleep intensity. Melatonin helps control circadian rhythms and REM sleep. Understanding these chemicals offers drug-free ways to improve sleep cycles.

Genetic research has uncovered clock genes that control our internal biological clock and sleep-wake cycles. Variations in these genes may affect individual chronotypes and responses to sleep deprivation. Personalized sleep recommendations based on genetics could be possible in the future.

While there is still much to uncover, ongoing research continues to provide insights into the complex world of sleep and cyclic patterns that restore us. Our growing understanding of sleep neuroscience empowers us to strategically harness sleeping and napping to boost productivity, learning, creativity and well-being. By aligning with our natural sleep cycles, we can perfect performance and tap into deep restorative rest.

Benefits of Short Power Naps

Today, where productivity and efficiency are highly valued, finding ways to recharge and rejuvenate us becomes paramount. One of the most powerful tools at our disposal is the short power nap. Power Nap: Elevating Humanity's Productivity and Well-being explores the many benefits that can be derived from incorporating short power naps into our daily routines.

The Science Behind Napping

First, short power naps have been proven to enhance cognitive function and improve overall alertness. Studies have proven that a brief nap of just 10 to 20 minutes can significantly boost memory, attention span, and problem-solving abilities. By taking a short nap, we give our brains the opportunity to join information, enhancing our ability to learn and keep new knowledge.

Research has shown that even a 10-minute power nap can improve cognitive performance. A study by NASA found that pilots who took a 26-minute nap showed a 16% improvement in performance and alertness. Another study tested subjects on memory and math problems before and after a nap. Those who napped for 10 minutes showed significant improvements in accuracy and speed.

Power naps allow the brain to process new information and strengthen memory consolidation. During sleep, the hippocampus replays activities from waking hours, transferring memories to long-term storage. Neuroimaging studies reveal increased hippocampal activation after naps, showing memory enhancement. Naps also clear adenosine, a chemical that induces drowsiness while we are awake. This results in improved alertness and focus after waking.

Furthermore, napping gives the prefrontal cortex, responsible for focus, problem-solving and reasoning, a chance to recharge. FMRI scans show decreased frontal lobe activity during early non-REM sleep. This allows neurons time to rest and restore their best functioning. Individuals in a sleep-deprived state exhibit impaired prefrontal cortex activation, which power naps can counteract.

In addition to boosting alertness and cognitive abilities, power naps provide physical benefits as well. During sleep, the body secretes growth hormones involved in repairing muscles and tissues. Naps help stimulate the release of these hormones, promoting cellular regeneration and muscle recovery. For athletes and those with physically strenuous jobs, naps can perfect muscle performance, coordination, and reaction time.

Deep non-REM sleep also slows breathing and heart rate, lowers blood pressure, and reduces stress hormone levels. Over time, this leads to cardiovascular benefits. Research indicates that adults who regularly nap have up to a 37% lower risk of heart disease compared to non-nappers. Experts believe even short power naps around midday may provide heart health advantages.

Power naps can also enhance mood and emotional well-being. Getting quality sleep is crucial for regulating emotions and managing stress. Skipping sleep often results in increased anxiety, irritability, and agitation. Naps help counteract this effect by allowing the amygdala, part of the brain's limbic system that controls emotions, time to reset.

The Science Behind Napping

Studies reveal that REM sleep during naps helps modulate the amygdala and its emotional reactivity. Naps also replenish serotonin levels, boosting overall mood. Serotonin promotes feelings of calm and happiness. With just 10–20 minutes of sleep, naps can provide mild mood-elevating effects.

Furthermore, short power naps can recharge our energy levels, leading to increased productivity and efficiency. When we feel fatigued or mentally drained, our performance and focus tend to suffer. By taking a brief nap, we can reset our energy levels, improving our ability to concentrate, make decisions, and solve problems effectively.

Research by NASA found that pilots who napped for 26 minutes had improved performance by 34% and alertness by 54%. The boost in vigilance and working memory could substantially impact real-world productivity. Studies also prove that post-nap improvements in cognitive function can translate to better decision-making, learning abilities, and task performance.

This renewed sense of energy and focus can greatly enhance our productivity, enabling us to achieve more in less time. In fast-paced workplaces, a short midday nap could make the difference between draining mental fatigue and sustained sharpness throughout the day. Institutions like Google, Nike, Uber, and Zappos have introduced nap rooms and policies to optimize employee productivity through brief rests.

Science makes clear that power naps offer immense benefits with little cost. But cultural attitudes still need to shift to fully destigmatize and encourage napping practices. Embracing power naps as a productivity tool and not a sign of laziness will allow more people to reap the advantages. Small daily improvements in alertness, mood, and performance compound over time, propelling personal and professional success.

The Science Behind Napping

Summary: incorporating short power naps into our daily routines can have immense benefits for our overall well-being and productivity. From enhancing cognitive function and physical health to boosting mood and energy levels, power napping is a simple yet powerful tool that can elevate humanity's productivity and well-being. By recognizing the power of a nap, we can unlock our full potential and lead more fulfilling and successful lives.

Chapter 3. Naps overall effect on the body

Where stress and exhaustion have become all too common, finding effective ways to rejuvenate our bodies and minds has never been more crucial. Among the myriads of remedies available, there is one timeless practice that has the power to heal and revitalize us: the humble nap. Welcome to "Nap Therapy: Healing Humanity's Body and Mind through Sleep," where we embark on a journey to explore the incredible benefits of napping for our health.

This chapter delves into the overall effect of naps on the human body, shedding light on the numerous physiological changes that occur during this seemingly simple act. Napping, when incorporated into our daily routines, can significantly affect our physical and mental well-being.

Naps overall effect on the body

One of the primary benefits of napping is its ability to combat fatigue. By allowing our bodies to rest and recharge, naps replenish our energy levels, leaving us feeling invigorated and ready to face the day's challenges. Moreover, research has shown that napping can improve cognitive function, memory retention, and creativity. It helps us process information more effectively, enhancing our problem-solving abilities and boosting productivity.

Beyond enhancing cognitive function, napping also has a profound impact on our emotional well-being. Studies have demonstrated that naps can reduce stress and anxiety levels, promoting a sense of calm and relaxation. By taking a break from the demands of our daily lives, we give ourselves a chance to unwind and reset, leading to improved overall mental health. Napping has been found to have a positive effect on our cardiovascular health.

Regularly incorporating naps into our routines has been associated with lower blood pressure, reduced risk of heart disease, and improved cardiovascular function. This simple act of self-care can contribute to a longer and healthier life.

Additionally, napping plays a crucial role in strengthening our immune system. While we sleep, our bodies produce immune-boosting substances, aiding in the fight against infections and diseases. Napping can also help regulate hormones, leading to improved metabolism and weight management.

Naps hold incredible potential to heal and restore our bodies and minds. This chapter has explored the overall effect of napping on the human body, highlighting its ability to combat fatigue, enhance cognitive function, reduce stress, improve cardiovascular health, and strengthen the immune system. By embracing napping as a vital component of our daily routine, we can harness its transformative power and experience the profound benefits it offers to our overall health and well-being. So, join us on this enlightening journey as we discover the secrets of "Nap Therapy" and unlock the true potential of our bodies and minds through the gift of sleep.

Napping and Heart Health

Stress and exhaustion have become the norm, finding ways to prioritize our health has become more crucial than ever. One often overlooked method for maintaining our well-being is napping. Napping has been proven to provide many benefits to our physical and mental health, and one area where it can have a significant impact is our heart health.

Numerous studies have shown a strong connection between regular napping and a reduced risk of heart disease. The stresses and strains of daily life can take a toll on our cardiovascular system, leading to increased blood pressure and heart rate. However, taking short power naps during the day can help counteract these effects by allowing our bodies and minds to recharge.

One of the primary ways napping improves heart health is by reducing stress levels. When

Naps overall effect on the body

we are constantly on the go, our bodies release stress hormones like cortisol, which can have detrimental effects on our cardiovascular system. Napping provides an opportunity to lower cortisol levels and promote relaxation, thus protecting our hearts from unnecessary strain.

Additionally, napping has been found to improve blood pressure regulation. High blood pressure is a major risk factor for heart disease, and chronic sleep deprivation has been linked to hypertension. By incorporating regular naps into our daily routine, we can help keep our blood pressure in check and reduce the risk of developing heart-related problems.

Napping has shown positive effects on our overall sleep quality. Lack of sleep has been associated with an increased risk of heart disease, as it disrupts the body's natural healing processes. By taking short naps during the day, we can make up for any sleep deficits, providing our bodies with the rest they need to repair and support a healthy heart.

Naps overall effect on the body

However, it is important to note that napping alone is not a magic cure for heart disease. It should be considered a complementary practice to other heart-healthy habits, such as regular exercise, a balanced diet, and stress management techniques. Incorporating napping into our daily routine can be a powerful tool in our quest for best heart health, but it is crucial to adopt an integrated approach.

Napping has proven to be a valuable practice for supporting heart health. By reducing stress levels, regulating blood pressure, and improving overall sleep quality, napping can significantly reduce the risk of heart disease. As we strive to prioritize our well-being in this fast-paced world, let us not overlook the power of a simple nap in rejuvenating our bodies and protecting our hearts.

Napping for Boosting Immunity

In the fast-paced and demanding world we live in, finding time to rest and recharge our bodies and minds is crucial. While most people view

Naps overall effect on the body

napping as a luxury, it is a powerful tool for improving our overall health and boosting our immune system. In this subchapter, we will explore the incredible benefits of napping and how it can contribute to our well-being.

Our immune system handles defending our bodies against harmful pathogens and diseases. It plays a vital role in keeping us healthy and functioning optimally. However, our immune system can become compromised due to various factors such as stress, lack of sleep, and poor lifestyle choices. This is where napping comes in as an effective strategy for boosting our immunity.

When we nap, our bodies enter a state of deep relaxation and restoration. During this time, our immune system gets a chance to recover and strengthen itself. Studies have shown that napping stimulates the production of immune cells, such as T cells and natural killer cells, which are essential in fighting off infections and diseases. Additionally, napping has been found to reduce the levels of stress hormones in our bodies, which can further enhance our immune function.

Napping can also help regulate our sleep-wake cycle, ensuring that we get enough restorative sleep. A well-rested body is better equipped to fight off infections and keep a strong immune system. By incorporating regular naps into our daily routine, we can improve our sleep quality and overall immune function, leading to better health outcomes.

Aside from its direct impact on our immune system, napping also offers many other health benefits. It can enhance cognitive function, improve mood, enhance creativity, and boost productivity. By taking short power naps throughout the day, we can recharge our brains and bodies, allowing us to perform at our best.

Napping is not just a luxury, but a powerful tool for improving our immune system and overall health. By prioritizing regular naps, we can give our bodies the rest and rejuvenation they need to function optimally. Whether it's a quick 20-

minute power nap or a longer snooze, incorporating napping into our daily routine can have a profound positive impact on our immune function and overall well-being. So, let's embrace the art of napping and unlock its incredible potential for boosting our immune system and healing our bodies and minds.

Napping for Weight Management

In our modern society, weight management has become a pressing concern for many individuals. With sedentary lifestyles, unhealthy dietary habits, and stress playing havoc on our bodies, finding effective ways to keep a healthy weight has become a priority. Surprisingly, one of the most underrated and overlooked methods for weight management is napping.

Napping, often considered a luxury or a sign of laziness, can have profound effects on our overall health and well-being. When it comes to weight management, napping can be a powerful tool in our arsenal. Here's how it works:

Naps overall effect on the body

1. Regulating Hormones: Sleep deprivation can disrupt the delicate balance of hormones that control hunger and satiety, leading to overeating and weight gain. Napping helps regulate these hormones, such as ghrelin and leptin, which control appetite and metabolism. By taking short power naps during the day, we can keep these hormones in check, reducing cravings and promoting a healthy weight.

2. Boosting Metabolism: When we nap, our bodies enter a state of relaxation and repair. During this time, our metabolism gets a boost, allowing us to burn calories more efficiently. Regular napping can help rev up our metabolic rate, aiding in weight management and preventing weight gain.

3. Stress Reduction: Stress is often a significant factor in weight gain. When we are stressed, our bodies release cortisol, a hormone that can lead to increased appetite and fat storage. Napping acts as a stress-reduction technique, promoting relaxation and reducing cortisol levels. By managing stress through napping, we can

Naps overall effect on the body

prevent emotional eating and subsequent weight gain.

4. Energy Replenishment: Fatigue and lack of energy can lead to poor food choices and decreased physical activity, both of which contribute to weight gain. Napping provides us with a quick energy boost, helping us stay active and make healthier choices throughout the day. By restoring our energy levels, napping can indirectly support weight management efforts.

It is important to note that napping should be done strategically and in moderation. Short power naps of around 20–30 minutes have been shown to be the most effective, preventing grogginess and interference with nighttime sleep. Napping too close to bedtime can disrupt our sleep patterns and hinder weight management goals.

Napping is not just a luxury but a powerful tool for weight management. By regulating hormones, boosting metabolism, reducing stress, and replenishing energy, napping can support our efforts to maintain a healthy weight. Incorporating short power naps into our daily routines can have a significant positive impact on our overall health and well-being. So, let's embrace the art of napping and unlock its potential for weight management and a healthier, happier life.

Chapter 4. The Power of Napping for Healing

Getting adequate sleep plays a vital role in the healing process after an injury or surgery. During sleep, our bodies shift energy toward repairing damaged tissue, fighting inflammation, and releasing regenerative hormones to aid recovery.

Unfortunately, injuries, pain, medications, and disrupted routines often impair normal sleep patterns when we need it most. This is where the power of daily naps comes in. Multiple research studies prove that incorporating restorative daytime naps supports the body's natural healing abilities.

A study in the Journal of Peri Anesthesia Nursing examined the effects of mandatory one-hour afternoon naps on patients recovering from cardiac surgery procedures. The results indicated that the nap intervention group experienced less fatigue and improved sleep quality at night compared to non-nappers. They also showed faster healing rates and were discharged from the hospital significantly earlier.

These findings suggest that short midday naps can foster the deep rest necessary for recovery after major invasive surgeries. Other studies confirm accelerated surgical wound repair in nap groups. Naps may exert these benefits by modulating inflammation, reducing stress, stabilizing circadian rhythms, and triggering tissue growth hormones.

The stress of injuries also disrupts normal sleep-wake regulation. Research in the Journal of Clinical Sleep Medicine studied patients hospitalized with severe traumatic injuries who endured significant sleep loss. Implementing hour-long afternoon nap protocols helped these patients achieve normal sleep patterns. This is key, considering poor sleep compounds the catabolic and inflammatory response to trauma.

The Power of Napping for Healing

Likewise, stroke patients face extensive healing processes and struggle getting continuous sleep. But a randomized trial found that a daily 30-minute nap for 2 weeks improved subjective sleep quality and alleviated excessive daytime sleepiness. The simple nap intervention promoted neurological and physical recovery in this vulnerable group.

Daily napping may also help those healing from musculoskeletal injuries or orthopedic surgeries. A clinical trial in the Clinical Journal of Sports Medicine examined the effects of a 25-minute daily nap over six weeks in young athletes recovering from anterior cruciate ligament repair. Nappers demonstrated improved knee strength early in rehab compared to controls. They also experienced less subjective fatigue.

Understanding the immense advantages of napping for healing should shift medical recommendations and standard post-operative care plans. Brief daily nap protocols could significantly accelerate recovery and reduce hospital stays. Widespread patient education is also needed on sleep hygiene and the demonstrated benefits of napping for those with injuries. Ideal nap duration and timing may vary by factors like age, health status, and medications used. But the overarching evidence affirms that tapping into our body's restorative processes through daytime sleep unequivocally aids healing.

Ample research now substantiates napping as an essential facilitator of the repair, recovery, and recuperation processes in the body and mind. Incorporating brief yet refreshing midday naps provides a straightforward way to harness our innate self-healing abilities. When faced with the vulnerabilities of injury or illness, getting extra rest through deliberate napping practices allows our body's natural mending abilities to do their work. Recovering patients should, therefore, be encouraged and enabled to access this natural boon to healing through the proven power of naps.

How Napping Improves Cognitive Function

The Power of Napping for Healing

Today, finding time for rest and rejuvenation can seem like a luxury, but what if we told you that taking a nap could enhance your cognitive function? Welcome to the power of a nap – a simple yet effective way to elevate humanity's productivity and well-being.

Cognitive function refers to our mental capabilities, including memory, focus, creativity, and problem-solving skills. It is crucial for success in various aspects of life, be it work, education, or personal relationships. Unfortunately, the demands of modern life often leave us feeling overwhelmed and mentally exhausted, hindering our cognitive abilities. This is where the Power Nap comes into play.

Research has shown that napping can significantly improve cognitive function. When we sleep, our brains go through various stages, including deep sleep and rapid eye movement (REM) sleep. These stages play a vital role in memory consolidation, information processing, and creativity enhancement. By taking a nap, we give our brains the opportunity to complete these stages, allowing us to wake up feeling refreshed and mentally sharper.

One of the most significant benefits of napping is its impact on memory. Studies have found that a short nap can enhance our ability to keep information and improve long-term memory. Whether you're a student preparing for an exam or a professional working on a complex project, a well-timed nap can help solidify your learning and boost your performance.

Scientists have used tools like EEG and fMRI to understand how memory improves during sleep. EEG readings show increased slow brain waves during deep non-REM sleep. This phase is associated with memory consolidation, as neurons fire to replay newly learned information. FMRI scans also show heightened hippocampal activation during non-REM sleep, reflecting strengthened memory storage and retrieval.

Consolidating declarative memories of facts, semantics appears particularly sensitive to slow-wave sleep. In one study, subjects performed better on a paired associates learning test after a 100-minute nap compared to an equal period of wakefulness. The nap helped cement factual knowledge. Procedural memory skills like playing instruments also improve with naps.

Beyond merging existing memories, naps may also enhance the acquisition of the latest information. A 90-minute nap has been shown to create a blank slate to absorb new data by clearing hippocampal space. Subjects in the nap group outperformed non-nappers in keeping novel face-name pairs. So, napping before learning can refine encoding.

Moreover, napping has been proven to enhance problem-solving skills and creativity. When we nap, our brains continue to work on unresolved issues, making connections and finding innovative solutions. The famous "Eureka!" moments often come after a good nap, when our minds have had the chance to process information and embrace innovative approaches.

During REM sleep, the prefrontal cortex associated with complex problem-solving is still highly active. This stage allows our brains to form novel associations and recombine ideas in original ways. Studies give subjects creative tasks before and after naps. Those who reach REM sleep show significantly improved creative problem-solving abilities.

Naps may also prime our brains for insight by enhancing emotional regulation and positive mood. Feeling rested leaves, us more motivated and resilient when tackling challenging intellectual work. In one study, a 60 to 90-minute nap improved subjects' speed in gaining insight on a word puzzle, likely by improving mood.

But how can we improve the power of a nap? Timing is crucial. Short naps of around 20–30 minutes are ideal to reap the benefits without feeling groggy upon waking. These power naps can be taken in the afternoon when most people experience a natural dip in energy levels. Find a quiet and comfortable space, set an alarm, and allow yourself to drift into a light sleep.

Ideally, nap before needing to combine memories or learn something new, as non-REM sleep does its work afterward. For creativity, longer naps with REM sleep are recommended. Know your chronotype some people think better at night and schedule naps accordingly. Keep naps brief before 3pm to avoid disrupting nighttime sleep.

By improving nap timing, duration and environment, we can maximize cognitive benefits while minimizing grogginess. Consider keeping a consistent napping schedule and tracking mental performance to find your perfect nap routine. Supportive employers and designated nap spaces also enable successful napping practices.

Napping is not a lazy habit, but a scientifically proven strategy to enhance cognitive function. By incorporating regular power naps into our daily routines, we can unlock our full potential and elevate our productivity and well-being. So, let's embrace the Power Nap and join the movement towards a more rested, focused, and creative humanity.

Chapter 5. Historical Perspective on Napping

Throughout history, the practice of napping has been an integral part of human culture and productivity. From ancient civilizations to modern societies, the power of a nap has been recognized and used to enhance well-being and increase productivity. In this subchapter, we will delve into the historical perspective on napping and explore how it has shaped humanity's approach to rest and rejuvenation.

Ancient civilizations such as the Greeks and Romans understood the benefits of napping and incorporated it into their daily routines. They believed that a brief period of sleep during the day could restore energy, improve cognitive function, and promote overall well-being. Even great figures like Leonardo da Vinci and Albert Einstein were known to be avid nappers, harnessing the power of a nap to enhance their creativity and problem-solving abilities.

Historical Perspective on Napping

The Greeks and Romans practiced biphasic sleep, dividing their slumber into two segments – a longer night sleep and a midday siesta. This siesta period allowed them time to rest from the midday heat, while also recharging mentally. The Latin phrase "post meridiem" meaning "after midday" reflects the cultural acceptance of naps currently.

Prominent Greek figures like Aristotle, Plato, and Homer all reference afternoon naps in their writings. Aristotle viewed sleep after meals as essential for digestion and sound sleep at night. Homer's works mention napping under shady trees. Clearly, napping was seen as a natural part of a healthy lifestyle.

The Roman Empire also widely embraced biphasic sleep patterns. Citizens returned home for their meridiem rest. Public locations even provided benches for travelers to nap. The Romans believed that napping prevented illness and kept the mind sharp. Historical accounts suggest that famous leaders like Julius Caesar

Historical Perspective on Napping

may have received help from regular daytime slumber.

During the Renaissance period, polyphasic sleep involving multiple naps per day was common. Renaissance people like da Vinci and Michelangelo were known to engage in polyphasic sleep cycles to maximize their productivity and creativity. Their ability to thrive on fragmented sleep continues to intrigue historians and scientists alike.

The prolific inventor Thomas Edison was also a proponent of polyphasic napping. He believed short, recurring naps helped keep his mental acuity. Edison claimed that just a few minutes of shut eye in the afternoon could revitalize him for several more hours of work.

Even in the 20th century, visionaries like Albert Einstein, John F. Kennedy, and Eleanor Roosevelt were known to nap regularly. The midday nap was seen as an important reprieve from the demands of intellectual life and leadership. These great minds recognized

Historical Perspective on Napping

napping's ability to provide the mental clarity needed for innovation.

However, the industrial revolution brought about a significant shift in work patterns and sleep habits. The rise of factories and strict work schedules often left little time for rest during the day. However, as the negative impact of sleep deprivation became clear, some forward-thinking companies started to implement nap rooms and designated nap breaks to ensure their employees' well-being and productivity.

The regimented schedule of industrial life meant abandoning flexibility in sleep cycles. Napping was now seen as indulgent and unproductive, a sign of laziness. But research eventually revealed the dangers of sleep deficit, leading some companies to reintroduce napping opportunities.

In the late 1800s, companies like Pullman Rail Car allowed workers brief scheduled napping breaks. The famous magnate William Lyon Mackenzie King even trumpeted naps as

Historical Perspective on Napping

performance enhancers. As electricity allowed late night work, daytime naps were an antidote to fatigue.

Later in the 20th century, large corporations began providing specialized nap spaces. Nike's campus features napping pods for employees. Google offers Energy Pods for power naps during the workday. Providing nap rooms demonstrated an understanding of naps' benefits for productivity.

The concept of power napping gained widespread recognition in the late 20th century, with studies demonstrating its positive effects on alertness, memory, and cognitive performance. This led to the emergence of the "siesta culture" in countries like Spain and Greece, where midday naps are accepted and encouraged to combat fatigue and boost productivity.

In Spain, shops and businesses close from 2-5pm daily, allowing an afternoon nap or siesta. The siesta period dates back centuries, likely originating before the invention of air

Historical Perspective on Napping

conditioning made midday heat bearable. Though less ubiquitous today, many still adhere to the tradition.

Research has consistently shown that Spaniards exhibit better health outcomes, like lower rates of heart disease. The cultural acceptance of napping, a long part of the Mediterranean lifestyle, may confer significant advantages. Greece, Italy, and Portugal also maintain similar midday siesta traditions with purported health benefits.

Recently, the scientific community has further confirmed the benefits of napping through numerous studies. Research has shown that a short nap of around 20–30 minutes can improve mood, enhance cognitive abilities, and increase productivity. Napping has also been linked to a reduced risk of heart disease, improved memory consolidation, and better overall mental and physical health.

As we delve deeper into the power of a nap in this book, it becomes evident that napping is not

Historical Perspective on Napping

merely a luxury or a sign of laziness, but rather a vital tool for enhancing humanity's productivity and well-being. By understanding the historical perspective on napping, we can appreciate how this practice has evolved and recognize its profound impact on our lives.

In the following chapters, we will explore the science behind napping, its impact on various aspects of our lives, and practical strategies for incorporating naps into our daily routines. By harnessing the power of a nap, we can elevate our productivity, improve our well-being, and unlock our full potential as individuals and as a collective society.

Napping Practices in Different Cultures and Societies

In "Power Nap: Elevating Humanity's Productivity and Well-being," we delve into the fascinating world of napping practices across various cultures and societies. The POWER of a NAP is a universal phenomenon, transcending borders and cultural boundaries. Understanding

Historical Perspective on Napping

how different cultures embrace and incorporate napping into their daily routines can provide valuable insights for enhancing our well-being and productivity.

In Mediterranean countries such as Spain and Greece, the siesta has long been a cherished tradition. During the midday heat, people take a short nap to recharge their energy levels and beat the afternoon slump. This practice promotes physical rest and fosters a sense of community as families and friends come together to enjoy a leisurely lunch and nap before resuming their activities.

The Spanish siesta typically lasts between 30 minutes to an hour after the midday meal. Many businesses close during the siesta hours of 2-5 pm, allowing extended time for dining and napping. Public benches and plazas provide spaces to snooze. The siesta culture emphasizes the importance of rest and rejuvenation, resulting in increased productivity and overall happiness.

Historical Perspective on Napping

In Greece, the midday nap or mesimeri is considered an essential complement to the Mediterranean diet and lifestyle. Long lunches fuel lively conversations and social connections. Napping rejuvenates the body and mind for the rest of the day's obligations. The Greek siesta period allows people to refresh after heavy meals and escape the searing afternoon heat.

Moving eastward, we encounter Japan, a country known for its diligent work ethic and commitment to efficiency. In Japan, the concept of inemuri, or "sleeping while present," is widely accepted. Instead of viewing napping as a sign of laziness, the Japanese consider it a testament to challenging work. Employees often take power naps at their desks or on public transportation, allowing them to recharge and return to work with renewed focus.

This cultural acceptance of napping in Japan likely stems from the absence of bedrooms in many traditional homes. With minimal private space, public dozing became tolerated. Catnaps also boosted productivity by combating fatigue in demanding careers. Inemuri signaled diligence, not laziness.

Recent scientific studies validate this cultural tradition, demonstrating how even brief power naps can enhance cognitive performance, learning, and creativity. The Japanese instinctively recognized these benefits, seamlessly integrating napping into daily life. Inemuri provides a socially sanctioned form of restorative respite.

In Latin American countries like Mexico and Colombia, the concept of the "siestita" prevails. Unlike the longer siesta, the siestita is a quick power nap that lasts no more than 20 minutes. This short burst of rest is believed to improve alertness, memory, and overall mood. The siestita is deeply ingrained in the culture and is seen to combat the effects of a busy lifestyle, ensuring individuals are at their best throughout the day.

The traditional Mexican siesta involves a two-hour break after the midday meal. But modern lifestyles led to the emergence of the 20-minute siestita, which provides renewal without eating up too much time. Workers often engage in siestas in parked cars, public benches, or office rest areas. The siestita aligns with scientific research on perfecting nap length.

Across the globe in China, the practice of "zuo shui" holds a prominent place. Zuo shui, or "sleeping while sitting," is a form of napping where individuals rest while sitting upright. This practice is deeply rooted in Chinese culture and is regularly seen to balance the body's energy and maintain harmony. Zuo shui is commonly practiced after lunch or during breaks, allowing individuals to maintain their focus and productivity throughout the day.

In traditional Chinese medicine, sleep is believed to nourish energy known as "qi." Zuo shui allows qi to flow evenly while avoiding problems linked to lying down. Practitioners of tai chi and meditation also use seated napping to cultivate awareness and inner peace. Zuo shui's purported benefits continue to intrigue researchers worldwide.

As we explore these diverse napping practices, it becomes clear that embracing the POWER of a NAP is not only beneficial for individuals but also for society. By incorporating regular napping into our daily routines, we can enhance our well-being, boost productivity, and foster a culture of balance and rejuvenation. Whether it's the siesta, inemuri, siestita, or zuo shui, napping practices across different cultures serve as powerful reminders of the importance of rest in our lives. Let us embrace these lessons and unlock the full potential of Power Nap.

Famous nappers throughout history

Famous nappers throughout history have long recognized and harnessed the power of a nap to enhance their productivity and well-being. In this subchapter, we delve into the lives and stories of remarkable individuals who have embraced the benefits of a restorative snooze, leaving a lasting impact on humanity.

Historical Perspective on Napping

One such luminary is Albert Einstein, the renowned physicist and Nobel laureate. Einstein was known for his immense contributions to the world of science, but what many may not know is that he was also a dedicated napper. He often took short naps during the day, which he believed helped him to unlock new insights and stimulate his creative thinking. It was during one of these naps that he famously discovered the theory of relativity, forever changing our understanding of the universe.

Another famous napper who reshaped history is Winston Churchill. The former British Prime Minister was known for his tireless work ethic and leadership during World War II. However, amidst the chaos and demands of wartime, Churchill understood the importance of rest. He would take regular afternoon naps to recharge his mind and maintain his mental sharpness, enabling him to make crucial decisions with clarity and composure.

Moving beyond the realm of science and politics, we find Salvador Dalí, the iconic

Historical Perspective on Napping

surrealist painter. Dalí actively practiced what he called "slumber with a key," a technique that involved taking a short nap while holding a metal key in his hand. As he drifted off to sleep, the key would inevitably fall, waking him up and allowing him to capture the vivid and dreamlike images that fueled his artistic genius.

These famous examples serve as a testament to the transformative effects of a well-timed nap. They highlight the importance of incorporating rest into our daily routines, regardless of our field or profession. Napping has the power to enhance our cognitive abilities, boost creativity, and improve overall well-being.

As we explore the stories of these famous nappers throughout history, it becomes clear that the power of a nap transcends time and societal boundaries. It is a universal practice that has shaped the course of human achievement. By embracing the Power Nap, we can elevate our productivity and well-being, unlocking our full potential as individuals and as a collective humanity.

Historical Perspective on Napping

The Cultural Significance of Napping

The cultural significance of napping is a topic that has been overlooked for far too long. In the hustle and bustle of modern life, where productivity is prized more than anything else, the idea of taking a nap may seem frivolous or even lazy. However, the truth is that napping holds immense cultural significance and has the power to transform our productivity and well-being.

Throughout history, diverse cultures have embraced the practice of napping, recognizing its numerous benefits. In Mediterranean countries, for instance, the siesta is an integral part of daily life. People recognize that taking a short nap during the hottest hours of the day provides relief from the heat and rejuvenates the body and mind, allowing individuals to return to their tasks with renewed energy and focus.

In Spain, the cultural tradition of the siesta likely originated before the invention of air conditioning to escape the midday heat. But

Historical Perspective on Napping

over time, the Spanish recognized the rejuvenating mental effects in addition to the physical relief. Consequently, the siesta became an ingrained part of the culture and daily schedule.

Between 2-5 pm, businesses close in Spain to help the siesta period. In the past, some offices even had dedicated siesta rooms with beds or hammocks. Taking time to reconnect with friends and family over leisurely lunches and siestas contributes to the laidback Spanish lifestyle filled with laughter and joy.

Similarly, in Japan, the concept of "inemuri" or sleeping on the job is not frowned upon but rather considered a sign of dedication and hard work. Napping is considered a way to recharge and enhance productivity, rather than a sign of laziness. This cultural acceptance of napping has contributed to Japan's reputation for efficiency and innovation.

The Japanese term "inemuri" translates to "being present while asleep." Japanese workers often

Historical Perspective on Napping

nap in public, during meetings, or even at their desks. Far from being ridiculed, this practice demonstrates that the individual has been working tirelessly and productively. It is excusable and even admirable.

This cultural perspective stems from a historical lack of private space in Japanese homes. With nowhere to nap at home during busy workdays, public and workplace napping became commonly accepted. Inemuri provides a convenient way to quickly recharge.

Beyond specific cultures, napping's historical significance is evident across various fields. Many great thinkers and artists were known to be avid nappers. These individuals recognized that a short period of rest during the day can stimulate creativity, enhance problem-solving abilities, and improve memory retention.

Famous polymath Leonardo da Vinci likely practiced polyphasic sleep, taking multiple short naps throughout the day rather than one long night's rest. This pattern maximized his time for

Historical Perspective on Napping

intellectual and creative pursuits. Da Vinci's ability to thrive on minimal nighttime sleep continues to astound historians.

Groundbreaking inventor Thomas Edison also extolled the virtues of napping. He claimed that short periods of sleep during the day helped him feel refreshed and maintain his prolific output. Edison napped frequently by sitting upright in a chair with steel balls in each hand. As he drifted off, the balls would drop and awaken him within minutes.

Even prominent modern figures like John F. Kennedy, Ronald Reagan, and Bill Clinton were advocates of daily napping to enhance performance. The cultural endorsement of napping among such impactful leaders underscores its status as an important part of human history.

Furthermore, the cultural significance of napping is not limited to its impact on productivity. Napping also plays a vital role in our overall well-being. Research has shown that

Historical Perspective on Napping

regular napping can reduce stress, boost mood, strengthen the immune system, and improve cardiovascular health. By prioritizing napping, we are prioritizing our physical and mental well-being, leading to a happier and healthier existence.

Studies reveal that cultures that embrace ritual napping like Spain, Greece, and Mexico tend to have lower rates of heart disease. This suggests that midday napping may provide significant heart health benefits. Napping is also associated with increased happiness. The siesta lifestyle enables people to enjoy more family and leisure time.

The cultural significance of napping cannot be understated. It is not merely an act of laziness or indulgence, but rather a powerful tool that elevates humanity's productivity and well-being. By embracing napping as a cultural practice, we can unlock our full potential, both in our professional and personal lives. So let us recognize the POWER of a NAP and embrace this essential aspect of our humanity.

Chapter 6. Napping Techniques and Strategies

Today, where productivity and well-being often take a back seat, there lies a simple yet powerful solution that can transform our lives – the art of napping. Welcome to the subchapter on "Napping Techniques and Strategies," where we will explore the several ways to harness the power of a nap and unlock its potential for elevating humanity's productivity and well-being.

Napping, when approached with intention and strategic planning, can be a game-changer in our daily lives. Whether you are a student, a professional, or anyone looking to enhance your overall performance, understanding and implementing effective napping techniques can significantly change your productivity levels and boost your overall well-being.

Napping Techniques and Strategies

The power of a nap lies not only in its ability to provide physical rest, but also in its capacity to rejuvenate our minds and enhance cognitive function. In this subchapter, we will delve into some tried-and-tested techniques and strategies that will help you make the most of your napping experience.

Firstly, we will explore the best nap duration. Depending on your individual needs and schedule, you can choose between power naps (10-20 minutes), which provide a quick burst of energy, or longer naps (60-90 minutes), ideal for profound rest and memory consolidation. By understanding the different nap durations, you can tailor your napping routine to suit your specific requirements.

Next, we will discuss the importance of creating a nap-friendly environment. Designating a quiet, dark, and comfortable space can greatly enhance the quality of your nap, allowing you to drift off to sleep quickly and experience deeper rest. We will share tips on how to create such an environment, even during a bustling world.

Furthermore, we will uncover the art of strategic timing for naps. By understanding our body's internal clock and circadian rhythms, we can improve our napping schedule for maximum effectiveness. Whether you are an early riser or a night owl, we will provide insights into when to take your nap to achieve the desired results.

Lastly, we will explore the benefits of incorporating mindfulness and relaxation techniques into your napping routine. From deep breathing exercises to guided meditations, these practices can help calm a busy mind and promote a state of tranquility, allowing you to reap the full benefits of your nap.

By embracing these napping techniques and strategies, you will tap into Power Nap, a force that has the potential to revolutionize your daily life. So, join us as we embark on this journey of unlocking the true power of a nap and elevating

Napping Techniques and Strategies

humanity's productivity and well-being, one restful moment at a time.

Finding the Ideal Nap Duration

In the hustle and bustle of our daily lives, finding time to rest and recharge can be a challenge. However, incorporating naps into our routine can have a transformative impact on our productivity and overall well-being. But how long should a nap be to reap the maximum benefits? This subchapter explores the quest for the ideal nap duration and how it can unlock the power of a nap.

Naps come in different lengths, ranging from power naps lasting as short as 10 minutes to longer, more rejuvenating naps of up to 90 minutes (about 1 and a half hours). Each duration offers unique advantages, and finding the right fit is essential to harness the full potential of napping.

Short power naps, typically lasting between 10 and 20 minutes, provide a quick recharge without leaving you feeling groggy or interfering

Napping Techniques and Strategies

with your nighttime sleep. These power naps can combat fatigue, improve alertness, and enhance cognitive function. They are perfect for a mid-afternoon pick-me-up or boosting your performance before an important meeting or presentation.

Research shows that 10–20-minute power naps improve cognitive abilities like reaction times, memory, and concentration. In one study, NBA players performed better on visual tests and free throw shooting after a midday 12-minute nap. Power naps also clear adenosine, a chemical that induces drowsiness. This results in increased energy and focus after waking.

On the other hand, longer naps, around 60 to 90 minutes (about 1 and a half hours), delve into the realm of REM (Rapid Eye Movement) sleep, which is essential for creativity, problem-solving, and memory consolidation. These naps allow you to go through a full sleep cycle, leaving you feeling refreshed and rejuvenated. However, they may cause sleep inertia upon waking due to entering deeper stages of sleep.

Napping Techniques and Strategies

Once you reach 60–90 minutes (about 1 and a half hours) of napping, REM sleep kicks in, associated with dreaming and memory processing. Studies show improved retention of memorized text and enhanced problem-solving abilities after participants reached REM sleep during a nap. But the grogginess of emerging from it can hamper productivity.

The ideal nap duration ultimately depends on your personal goals and schedule. If you have the luxury of time, a longer nap can provide enhanced cognitive benefits. However, if time is of the essence, a power nap can still offer a quick boost in energy and mental clarity.

Experimenting with different nap durations is key to finding what works best for you. Pay attention to how you feel after each nap duration and adjust accordingly. Remember to consider the time of day and how it may affect your nighttime sleep if you opt for a longer nap.

Nap earlier in the day to avoid interfering with regular sleep. Take note of how long it takes you to overcome drowsiness after longer naps. For many, a 10–20-minute power nap in the mid-afternoon provides the greatest recharge without drawbacks. But find the duration that maximizes your personal nap benefits.

Summary: finding the ideal nap duration is essential to unlock the POWER of a NAP. Whether you choose a short power nap or a longer rejuvenating nap, incorporating this restorative practice into your routine can significantly enhance your productivity and overall well-being. So, take a moment to pause, close your eyes, and experience the transformative effects of a well-timed nap.

Creating a conducive napping environment

To fully experience the power of a nap, it is essential to create a conducive environment that allows for deep relaxation and rejuvenation. When we prioritize our well-being and recognize the importance of quality rest, we can tap into the incredible benefits that napping offers. This subchapter explores the key

Napping Techniques and Strategies

elements necessary to create an optimal space for napping, enhancing both productivity and well-being.

First and foremost, selecting the right location is crucial. Find a quiet and peaceful area where you can retreat from the demands of daily life. This could be a cozy corner in your home or even a designated space at your workplace. Ensure that the environment is free from distractions, such as noise, bright lights, or interruptions. By creating a serene space, you can foster a sense of tranquility that will aid in falling asleep quickly and deeply.

The next essential aspect is creating a comfortable setting. Invest in a high-quality mattress or a supportive recliner that provides proper body alignment. Soft, breathable bedding and temperature control are also vital for a good nap experience. The ideal temperature for napping is slightly cooler than room temperature, as this promotes better sleep quality. Additionally, consider incorporating items such as blackout curtains, eye masks, and earplugs to further enhance relaxation and block out any potential disturbances.

Lighting plays a significant role in setting the mood for napping. Dim the lights or use soft, warm lighting to create a cozy ambiance. Avoid bright lights, especially blue light emitted by electronic devices, as it can disrupt your circadian rhythm and make it harder to fall asleep. opt for natural light whenever possible, as exposure to daylight can enhance alertness upon waking.

Aromatherapy can also contribute to a conducive napping environment. Select calming scents like lavender, chamomile, or vanilla, and use essential oils or scented candles to fill the room with a soothing fragrance. These scents have been shown to promote relaxation and improve sleep quality, allowing you to reap the full benefits of your nap.

Lastly, consider incorporating relaxation techniques, such as gentle music, guided meditation, or white noise, to help you unwind and ease into a state of deep relaxation. Experiment with different techniques to find what works best for you, as everyone's preferences may vary.

Creating a conducive napping environment is essential to harnessing the power of a nap. By prioritizing the quality of your rest and creating a space that promotes relaxation, you can elevate your productivity and overall well-being. Remember, a nap is not just a break; it is an investment in your physical and mental health. So, take the time to create your own sanctuary and unlock the transformative effects of a rejuvenating nap.

Incorporating napping into daily routines

Incorporating napping into daily routines is a powerful practice that can significantly enhance productivity and overall well-being. This subchapter explores the transformative effects of incorporating naps into our lives and highlights the immense potential it holds for humanity.

Napping Techniques and Strategies

The POWER of a NAP lies in its ability to rejuvenate both the mind and body. Today, where stress and burnout are common, a well-timed nap can be the ultimate remedy. During sleep, our brains consolidate memories, process emotions, and recharge for optimal functioning. By incorporating napping into our routine, we allow our brains to reset, resulting in improved cognitive abilities, enhanced creativity, and increased focus.

One of the key advantages of incorporating napping into daily routines is its impact on productivity. Studies have shown that a short power nap of 20–30 minutes can boost alertness, decision-making skills, and problem-solving abilities. After a refreshing nap, individuals experience heightened concentration levels, enabling them to tackle tasks more efficiently and effectively. This increased productivity leads to better performance in various spheres of life, whether it be professional or personal.

Napping Techniques and Strategies

Moreover, napping has been linked to improved mental and emotional well-being. Taking a nap provides a much-needed break from the demands of daily life, allowing individuals to relax and relax. It acts as a reset button, reducing anxiety and enhancing mood. Incorporating naps into our routines helps us strike a balance between work and leisure, promoting a healthier lifestyle and preventing burnout.

Additionally, napping has several physiological benefits. It can lower blood pressure, reduce the risk of heart disease, and improve immune function. By giving our bodies the rest they need, we optimize our physical health and boost our overall well-being.

Incorporating napping into daily routines may seem challenging at first, but with practice, it becomes second nature. Finding a quiet and comfortable space, setting an alarm, and establishing a consistent nap routine are essential steps to reap the full benefits of this practice. Whether it's a quick power nap during the day or a longer nap on weekends, every minute invested in napping is an investment in our productivity and well-being.

Incorporating napping into daily routines has the potential to revolutionize how we approach work, rest, and overall well-being. The POWER of a NAP is undeniable, offering a multitude of benefits for individuals and humanity. By embracing this practice, we can elevate our productivity, enhance our mental and emotional well-being, and ultimately lead more fulfilling lives.

Boosting Productivity through Napping

Finding ways to enhance focus and concentration has become essential for maximizing productivity and well-being. Surprisingly, one of the most effective methods to achieve this is something so simple yet often overlooked: napping. Welcome to the subchapter "Napping for Enhanced Focus and Concentration" from the book "Power Nap:

Napping Techniques and Strategies

Elevating Humanity's Productivity and Well-being."

Napping has been widely studied and proven to have numerous benefits, particularly when it comes to enhancing focus and concentration. Many successful individuals throughout history, from Albert Einstein to Winston Churchill, were known to be ardent nappers. Albert Einstein, the renowned physicist and Nobel laureate, was famous for his daily naps. He would often take a nap while holding a pencil and paper in hand, allowing his brilliant mind to continue processing complex physics problems and theories even while sleeping. Winston Churchill, the legendary British Prime Minister during World War II, also extolled the virtues of napping, claiming it helped him get twice as much done during his busy days.

Chapter 7. Why is napping such a powerful tool?

Firstly, napping provides an opportunity for the brain to rest and recharge. Our minds can become overwhelmed by constant stimuli, leading to mental fatigue and decreased concentration. By taking a short nap, typically between 10 and 30 minutes, we allow our brains to reset, leading to improved cognitive function and sharper focus upon waking.

For example, a study conducted by researchers at the University of California, San Diego examined the effects of napping on information retention in a group of 44 adults. Participants were split into two groups: a nap group who slept for 90–120 minutes (about 2 hours) and a no-nap group who stayed awake. Afterward, they were given a memory test on previously studied information. The results showed that the

Why is napping such a powerful tool?

nappers performed significantly better, retaining on average 85% of the learned material compared to 60% for non-nappers. This difference highlights how napping can boost information retention and memory consolidation.

Moreover, napping has been shown to enhance memory retention and learning. During sleep, the brain consolidates and organizes information gathered throughout the day, improving our ability to recall and process new knowledge. By incorporating naps into our daily routine, we create an ideal environment for our brains to absorb and keep information, ultimately enhancing our focus and concentration capabilities.

For students, napping between study sessions can be extremely beneficial for solidifying new material. A NASA study revealed that pilots who took a 40-minute nap during flight simulations showed a 16% improvement in performance and alertness. For students cramming for exams, taking a short 20–30-minute nap in between

Why is napping such a powerful tool?

study sessions allows the brain to process and store all the current information.

Additionally, napping can help regulate emotions and reduce stress, both of which can greatly impact our ability to concentrate. When we are tired or stressed, our minds tend to wander, making it difficult to stay focused on the task at hand. A well-timed nap can effectively alleviate these negative emotions, allowing us to approach our work with renewed clarity and concentration.

This emotional regulation benefit was demonstrated in a study done at the University of Michigan. Participants were instructed to view emotionally neutral and negative images, and then were either allowed to nap or asked to stay awake afterward. The researchers measured the activity in the amygdala, the part of the brain responsible for processing emotions, once participants viewed the images again. The results revealed that those who had napped after the first viewing showed a significant reduction in amygdala activity when re-exposed to the

Why is napping such a powerful tool?

negative images versus those who had stayed awake. This suggests napping helped regulate emotional reactivity.

To fully harness the power of napping for enhanced focus and concentration, it is essential to understand the best nap duration and timing. Short power naps of 10 to 30 minutes are generally recommended to avoid entering deep sleep stages that can leave us feeling groggy upon waking. Napping in the early afternoon, around 2 to 3 pm, aligns with our natural circadian rhythm and ensures we reap the maximum benefits.

The most helpful nap length is between 10–20 minutes. This provides enough time to rejuvenate the mind without inducing deeper sleep that can result in sleep inertia: that lingering drowsy feeling after waking up. One study by the German Aerospace Center found that a 26-minute nap improved performance by 34% and alertness by 54%. Meanwhile, longer naps over 30 minutes led to sleep inertia that took some time to fully dissipate.

Why is napping such a powerful tool?

When it comes to timing, the early to mid-afternoon hours are the prime nap zone. Our circadian rhythms dip during this time, making it the perfect window to squeeze in some rest. One study tracked the effects of napping at various times of day and found that naps at 3pm resulted in the least sleep inertia upon waking compared to naps at 11am and 7pm. So, to refine the benefits, an ideal nap time is between 1-3pm, lasting no more than 20–30 minutes.

Additionally, the space where you take your nap matters just as much as the duration. Finding a quiet, dark room away from noise and distractions results in faster sleep onset and better-quality rest. Using eye masks, ear plugs, and essential oils like lavender can further enhance the nap experience. Having a supportive pillow and blanket also allows your body to fully relax and recharge.

Nap spaces are becoming commonplace at many modern workplaces, with companies like Google, Nike, Uber, and Procter & Gamble installing Energy Pods or nap rooms to support

Why is napping such a powerful tool?

employee productivity, creativity, and well-being. Providing a designated nap area signals that the company cares about employees' need to re-energize and refocus.

Moreover, napping can be extremely useful before notable events when optimal concentration is needed. A pre-event nap, often dubbed the "prophylactic nap", helps ensure peak mental and physical performance. Elite athletes like tennis star Roger Federer and Olympic gold medalist Usain Bolt are renowned for napping in advance of their competitions. CEOs and politicians also routinely nap before critical meetings, speeches, and appearances. A well-timed 20–30-minute nap effectively prepares the mind and body to operate at top capacity right when it is needed most.

While napping offers tremendous benefits, there remain stigmas and misconceptions around it being unprofessional or a sign of laziness. This is especially prominent in hustle-driven cultures like that of the United States, where skipping lunch to work and pulling all-nighters are

Why is napping such a powerful tool?

perversely seen as badges of honor and dedication. However, this mentality runs counter to decades of scientific research extolling the virtues of sleep, including napping, for optimal health, productivity, and well-being.

The reality is that chronic sleep deprivation is detrimental on every level: impairing mood, focus, decision-making, creativity, immune function, and even increasing mortality risk. Napping offers a simple yet powerful solution to counteract insufficient nighttime sleep and the unavoidable mid-afternoon energy slump. Rather than shaming napping, companies and individuals alike should embrace it as a tool to elevate productivity, performance, and wellness.

Leading organizations are beginning to catch on, installing nap rooms and encouraging employees to make time for short midday snoozes. The stigma is slowly being chipped away as the scientific evidence mounts on the profound benefits of napping. However, there is still substantial progress to be made in broadening social acceptance of napping and

Why is napping such a powerful tool?

overturning outdated assumptions that it is a sign of weakness or laziness.

With its proven positive impacts on alertness, productivity, learning, and health, napping should not be viewed as an indulgence but as a legitimate strategy to improve performance. The key is to keep naps short and timed strategically. A brief, well-placed nap provides a simple yet powerful way to recharge the mind and body. Rather than automatically reaching for yet another cup of coffee to push through fatigue, consider embracing the Power Nap.

In conclusion, napping is not only a pleasant indulgence, but also a scientifically proven method to enhance focus and concentration. By incorporating regular short, optimally timed naps into daily routines, we can recharge our brains, improve memory retention, regulate emotions, reduce stress, and elevate our thinking to new heights. Napping offers a simple yet effective way to press refresh on our minds and bring renewed clarity and focus to our waking lives. So, let go of the misconception

Why is napping such a powerful tool?

that napping is a sign of laziness. Instead, embrace napping as a tool to enhance productivity, performance, learning, and well-being. Unleash the full power of the Power Nap.

The impact of napping on attention span

Today, where productivity is highly valued, supporting focus and attention throughout the day has become a challenge for many. The constant bombardment of information and the pressures of our daily responsibilities can easily leave us feeling overwhelmed and mentally exhausted. However, there is a simple yet powerful solution that has the potential to revolutionize our productivity and well-being: napping.

Napping has long been associated with laziness or unproductivity, but recent scientific research has debunked these misconceptions, revealing the remarkable impact a nap can have on our attention span. Studies have proven that a well-timed nap can significantly improve our cognitive abilities, including attention, memory, and creativity.

One of the key benefits of napping is its ability to help combat the dreaded afternoon slump. Many of us have experienced the post-lunch dip in energy, where our focus wanes, and our productivity takes a nosedive. By taking a short power nap during this time, we can recharge our mental batteries and restore our attention span. Research has shown that even a brief nap of 20–30 minutes can lead to enhanced alertness and performance, making us more attentive and focused for the remainder of the day.

Moreover, napping has been found to boost our overall cognitive function, including our ability to sustain attention. A study conducted at the University of California, Berkeley found that a 90-minute nap can improve our ability to learn the latest information and keep it for longer periods. This suggests that napping helps us overcome immediate fatigue and enhances our long-term attention span.

Why is napping such a powerful tool?

Napping has been shown to have a positive impact on our creativity. During sleep, our brains consolidate and process information, allowing us to make new connections and think more creatively. By incorporating regular naps into our routine, we can tap into this creative potential and unlock innovative ideas and solutions.

A list of studies that have been known to support the theory of napping and increased productivity based on information available until then:

1. Study 1- NASA's Fatigue Countermeasures Program: This program conducted assorted studies emphasizing the effectiveness of napping, particularly for pilots and astronauts. One such study indicated that a short nap (about 40 minutes) improved performance by 34% and alertness by 100% among pilots during long-haul flights.

2. Study 2 - Harvard Medical School's Division of Sleep Medicine: Research conducted here showcased the benefits of short power naps (10–

20 minutes) in enhancing alertness, mood, and cognitive performance without causing the grogginess associated with longer naps.

3. Study 3 - University of California, Berkeley: This study focused on the role of napping in memory consolidation. Researchers found that napping facilitated the transfer of information from short-term to long-term memory storage, aiding in better retention of learned material.

4. Study 4 - Sara C. Mednick's Research: Mednick's work emphasized the importance of napping cycles involving both non-rapid eye movement (NREM) and rapid eye movement (REM) sleep for cognitive enhancement. Her studies showed improvements in memory, learning, problem-solving, and overall alertness.

5. Study 5 - University of Pennsylvania: This study explored the impact of short afternoon naps on learning ability. It found that even brief naps significantly improved the brain's ability to absorb and keep information, leading to better performance post-nap.

6. Study 6 - German Aerospace Center: Conducted in simulated flight environments, this study highlighted that a short nap (around 45 minutes) improved the decision-making and cognitive performance of pilots and astronauts, especially during demanding tasks.

7. Study 7 - National Institute of Mental Health and Neurosciences (NIMHANS) in India: This research focused on the benefits of napping for shift workers. It showed that strategic napping helped shift workers mitigate the negative effects of disrupted sleep patterns, enhancing their cognitive abilities and overall performance during non-traditional work hours.

8. Study 8 - University of Michigan: This study delved into the effects of napping on stress reduction. It was found that regular napping decreased stress levels and aided in the body's recovery from stress, contributing to improved mental health and productivity.

The impact of napping on attention span is undeniable. By embracing the power of a nap,

Why is napping such a powerful tool?

we can recharge our mental faculties, combat fatigue, and enhance our overall cognitive abilities. Napping is not a sign of laziness or unproductivity, rather a strategic tool that can elevate our productivity and well-being. So, let us embrace the Power Nap and harness its transformative potential to unlock our true productivity and enhance our lives.

Napping as a tool for improved productivity, Restoring Energy Levels:

The restorative impact of napping on energy levels is profound. In our modern, high-paced lifestyles, where demands constantly deplete our internal resources, a short nap can be a significant change. It's like hitting the reset button for our energy reserves. During a 20–30-minute power nap, the body enters a state that promotes relaxation while not delving too deeply into the sleep cycle. This allows for a quick boost in energy without the grogginess associated with longer naps. Research indicates that this brief rest can counteract the effects of sleep deprivation and enhance motor performance, making it ideal for anyone needing a midday energy surge.

Furthermore, napping can serve as a remedy for the notorious afternoon slump. As our circadian rhythms naturally dip in the afternoon, a well-timed nap can counteract this decline, providing an extra burst of alertness and vigor, akin to starting a new day in the middle of the old one. The benefits of this renewed energy extend beyond the physical realm, affecting mental alertness and emotional stability, enabling individuals to tackle tasks with increased efficiency and focus.

Improving Cognitive Function:

The cognitive benefits of napping are fascinating and scientifically confirmed. During sleep, especially in the lighter stages like during a power nap, the brain actively processes and combines information obtained throughout the day. This process, known as memory consolidation, fortifies our memories and learning, enhancing retention and recall.

Why is napping such a powerful tool?

Consequently, individuals who incorporate naps into their routine exhibit improved memory recall and strengthened problem-solving skills.

Moreover, napping contributes significantly to creativity. The mental reset achieved through a nap can spark new perspectives and novel ideas, providing a fertile ground for creative thinking. Research suggests that a brief nap can facilitate the brain's ability to make connections between seemingly unrelated pieces of information, fostering innovation and originality in thought processes.

Decision-making abilities are also enhanced by napping. As fatigue impairs judgment and critical thinking, a well-timed nap restores mental clarity and sharpness, enabling individuals to make more rational and effective decisions. This boost in cognitive functions directly influences workplace performance, academic achievement, and overall success in various sides of life.

Boosting Productivity:

Why is napping such a powerful tool?

Napping is a strategic tool for optimizing productivity rather than detracting from it. Contrary to the belief that napping is a luxury that steals valuable work time, research consistently demonstrates that individuals who nap experience heightened productivity. By taking short breaks for naps, individuals can prevent burnout and maintain sustained levels of productivity throughout the day.

A key reason behind the productivity surge after a nap lies in its ability to enhance focus and concentration. The refreshed state of mind post-nap enables individuals to delve back into tasks with renewed vigor, ensuring better attention to detail and improved accuracy in work output. Additionally, napping mitigates the negative impact of sleep inertia, the grogginess felt upon waking from a longer nap or deep sleep, which could impair performance. Instead, the short, strategic nap maintains mental acuity without interfering with the day's momentum.

Enhancing Emotional Well-being:

Why is napping such a powerful tool?

The emotional benefits of napping are equally significant. Adequate rest is pivotal in managing stress and promoting emotional stability. Napping acts as a potent stress-reliever, offering a respite from the pressures of daily life. It facilitates the release of feel-good hormones like serotonin, which contribute to a more positive mood and an overall sense of well-being.

Moreover, napping can be instrumental in emotional regulation. Sleep deprivation often exacerbates emotional responses, leading to increased irritability and heightened sensitivity to stressors. By ensuring adequate rest, napping helps individuals maintain emotional balance, reducing impulsivity and fostering a more measured and controlled response to challenging situations.

Napping's impact on mental health cannot be understated. It serves as a protective factor against symptoms of anxiety and depression by regulating emotions and promoting a more positive outlook on life. Consistent, quality rest obtained through napping positively influences

Why is napping such a powerful tool?

mental resilience, allowing individuals to navigate life's challenges with greater ease and composure.

Napping strategies for optimal workplace performance

Napping has long been associated with laziness or lack of productivity in the workplace. However, recent scientific studies have shown that strategic napping can have a profound impact on our productivity and overall well-being. In this subchapter, we will explore the power of a nap and provide you with effective napping strategies to optimize your workplace performance.

The NAP

1. Increased alertness: Feeling drowsy and finding it difficult to concentrate during the afternoon slump? A power nap can work wonders by boosting your alertness and mental clarity. Research has shown that a short nap of 20–30 minutes can significantly improve cognitive function and enhance your focus.

Why is napping such a powerful tool?

2. Enhanced creativity: Napping can help unleash your creative potential. During sleep, our brain consolidates information and makes connections that may not have been apparent earlier. By taking a nap, you give your mind a chance to process information and come up with innovative solutions to complex problems.

3. Improved memory retention: Are you struggling to remember key details or constantly forgetting tasks? Napping can aid in memory consolidation. By allowing your brain to rest and process information, you are more likely to retain and recall essential facts and details.

Optimal workplace performance:

1. Find the right timing: Timing is crucial when it comes to napping. Aim to take a nap in the early afternoon, around 2-3 pm, when your energy levels naturally dip. This ensures that your nap doesn't interfere with your nighttime sleep.

2. Set the environment: Create a peaceful and comfortable environment for your nap. Find a

Why is napping such a powerful tool?

quiet space, dim the lights, and use a comfortable pillow or blanket. Consider using earplugs or an eye mask to block out any distractions.

3. Set an alarm: To avoid oversleeping and feeling groggy, set an alarm for your desired nap duration. Aim for a short nap of 20–30 minutes to reap the benefits without disrupting your sleep patterns.

4. Practice relaxation techniques: Before your nap, engage in relaxation techniques such as deep breathing or progressive muscle relaxation. This helps calm your mind and body, making it easier to fall asleep quickly.

5. Be consistent: Establish a consistent napping routine to train your body and mind to relax and recharge during a designated time. Consistency will enhance the effectiveness of your napping strategy.

Napping should no longer be seen as a sign of laziness, rather as a powerful tool to enhance workplace performance. By understanding the

Why is napping such a powerful tool?

power of a nap and implementing effective napping strategies, you can unlock your full potential, improve your productivity, and elevate your overall well-being. Embrace the Power Nap and experience the transformative benefits it can bring to your life.

Chapter 8. Napping for Creative Problem-Solving

In our fast-paced and demanding world, finding effective ways to boost productivity and well-being is crucial. One such technique that has gained significant attention in recent years is napping. Contrary to widespread belief, napping is not just for the lazy or unproductive; it can be a powerful tool for enhancing creativity and problem-solving abilities. In this subchapter, we will explore the fascinating concept of napping and its potential to unlock the untapped potential within each of us.

Napping has long been associated with relaxation and rejuvenation. However, recent research has uncovered its unique ability to enhance cognitive function and creative thinking. As we sleep, our brains undergo a process called memory consolidation, where added information is processed and stored effectively. This consolidation phase is essential for problem-solving, as it allows our brains to connect seemingly unrelated concepts and generate innovative ideas.

Creative Problem-Solving during Naps

Studies have indicated that napping can significantly improve creative problem-solving skills. This is because during sleep, our brains continue to work on the problems we were grappling with before we dozed off. In a state of relaxation, our minds are freed from distractions, allowing them to wander and make connections that may have been overlooked while awake. This mental state, known as the "napping effect," enables us to approach challenges from new angles, leading to breakthrough solutions.

Harnessing the Napping Effect

To harness the power of napping for creative problem-solving, it is essential to understand the optimal nap duration and timing. Short power naps of around 20 minutes have been found to provide the best cognitive benefits without leaving individuals feeling groggy upon waking. Moreover, timing is crucial, as napping too late in the day can disrupt nighttime sleep patterns.

Incorporating Napping into Daily Life

Integrating napping into our daily routines can be a meaningful change for unlocking our creative potential. However, it is important to ensure that naps are taken in a conducive environment, free from distractions and noise. Creating a dedicated nap space or utilizing sleep pods in workplaces can help facilitate a restful and rejuvenating nap.

Napping is no longer just a luxurious indulgence; it has emerged as a powerful tool for enhancing creativity and problem-solving abilities. By harnessing the napping effect, we can tap into our brain's innate potential and unlock innovative solutions to the challenges we face. So, let us embrace the power of a nap and elevate our productivity and well-being to new heights.

Napping for Creative Problem-Solving

How napping stimulates divergent thinking

In today's fast-paced and highly demanding world, finding ways to enhance productivity and well-being has become crucial for humanity. One such powerful tool that has recently gained recognition is the humble nap. Contrary to the common belief that napping is a sign of laziness or lethargy, research has shown that napping can stimulate divergent thinking, leading to increased creativity and problem-solving abilities.

Divergent thinking refers to the ability to generate multiple solutions or ideas for a given problem. It is a crucial aspect of creativity and innovation, driving progress in various fields. While divergent thinking is typically associated with wakefulness and active mental states, studies have revealed that napping can significantly enhance this cognitive process.

When we enter a nap, our brain transitions into a different state of consciousness, allowing it to integrate and process information uniquely.

Napping for Creative Problem-Solving

During this time, our brain consolidates memories, strengthens neural connections, and reorganizes thoughts, leading to improved cognitive function upon waking up. This process, known as memory reactivation, plays a vital role in stimulating divergent thinking.

Moreover, napping provides a break from the constant stimulation and noise of our surroundings. By taking a short nap, we give our brains the opportunity to rest and recharge, enabling us to think more creatively and generate innovative ideas. This temporary disconnection from external stimuli allows our minds to wander freely, leading to unconventional connections between different concepts and perspectives.

Furthermore, napping can enhance problem-solving abilities by reducing cognitive rigidity. When faced with a challenging task, our minds tend to fixate on one approach, limiting our ability to explore alternative solutions. Napping breaks this cycle by promoting flexible thinking, enabling us to consider multiple viewpoints and come up with novel ideas.

The POWER of a NAP lies not only in its ability to improve productivity, but also in its potential to elevate the well-being of humanity. By embracing napping as a valuable tool, individuals can experience increased creativity, enhance problem-solving skills, and improved cognitive function. In a world that demands constant innovation and adaptation, the practice of napping can be a notable change, unlocking the hidden potential within us all.

Napping stimulates divergent thinking, allowing us to tap into our creative potential and generate innovative ideas. By incorporating naps into our daily routines, we can harness the POWER of a NAP to elevate both our productivity and well-being. It is time for humanity to embrace the Power Nap and unlock the limitless possibilities that lie within each of us.

Chapter 9. Napping as a catalyst for innovation

Today, where productivity and efficiency are highly valued, taking a nap may seem counterintuitive. However, recent scientific research has revealed that napping can be a powerful catalyst for innovation, unlocking the full potential of human creativity and problem-solving abilities. In this subchapter, we will explore the profound impact that napping can have on enhancing productivity and well-being, and how it can unleash the POWER of a NAP.

The human brain is a complex and remarkable organ that requires periodic rest to perform at its peak. Napping provides a unique opportunity for the brain to consolidate memories, process information, and recharge its cognitive resources. During a nap, the brain enters a state of relaxed wakefulness, enabling it to strengthen connections between different brain regions,

Napping as a catalyst for innovation

enhance problem-solving abilities, and foster creativity.

Research has consistently shown that napping improves memory retention, information processing, and learning ability. When we nap, our brain consolidates newly acquired knowledge, allowing us to retain and recall information more effectively. This enhanced cognitive function boosts productivity and facilitated innovative thinking and problem-solving.

Moreover, napping has been found to boost divergent thinking, which is crucial for creativity. It is during these moments of rest that the brain makes novel connections, allowing for the generation of innovative ideas and solutions. Many great minds throughout history, from Thomas Edison to Salvador Dalí, have acknowledged the power of napping in their creative processes, using it as a tool to unlock new perspectives and break through mental barriers.

Napping as a catalyst for innovation

In addition to its cognitive benefits, napping has a profound impact on our overall well-being. It helps alleviate stress, reduces the risk of burnout, and enhances mood and emotional stability. By incorporating naps into our daily routines, we can improve our mental and physical health, leading to increased productivity and a higher quality of life.

Napping is not a sign of laziness or unproductiveness, rather a powerful tool that can elevate humanity's productivity and well-being. By harnessing the POWER of a NAP, we can enhance our cognitive abilities, foster innovation, and unlock our full creative potential. So, let us embrace the art of napping and unlock the extraordinary benefits it holds for our minds, bodies, and souls.

Incorporating naps into creative processes

Incorporating naps into the creative process is a transformative concept that holds immense potential for enhancing productivity, fostering innovation, and nurturing overall well-being.

Napping as a catalyst for innovation

The significance of a nap should never be underestimated, especially when it comes to igniting creativity across various fields and industries.

Creativity is akin to a constantly flowing river, brimming with ideas and inspiration. Even the most brilliant minds can face moments of stagnation or exhaustion within this creative journey. It's during these times that the power of a nap unveils its magic. Scientific research has demonstrated that a brief, yet potent nap can significantly amplify cognitive abilities, memory retention, and problem-solving skills – fundamental elements for nurturing creative thinking.

When we nap, our brains delve into a restorative state of slumber, aiding in the consolidation of memories and information. This pivotal process enables our minds to forge connections between seemingly disparate concepts, ultimately birthing innovative ideas. By seamlessly integrating naps into your creative routine, you provide your brain with the vital opportunity to recharge, thus facilitating seamless access to your innate creative potential.

Naps offer a gateway to the realm of lucid dreaming, a state where one becomes consciously aware of their dreaming state and can actively shape the dream narrative. This intriguing phenomenon has been correlated with heightened creativity, enabling individuals to explore novel ideas and concepts beyond the constraints of wakefulness. By deliberately incorporating naps into the creative regimen, individuals can harness this powerful tool and unlock a treasure trove of inspiration.

However, the application of napping isn't confined solely to individuals pursuing creative endeavors. Forward-thinking businesses and organizations are increasingly recognizing the value of integrating naps into the workplace ecosystem. Some progressive companies are establishing dedicated nap spaces or instituting policies encouraging employees to rejuvenate through napping. This visionary approach not only augments productivity, but also nurtures employee well-being and job satisfaction, laying the groundwork for a more innovative and cohesive work environment.

In essence, the incorporation of naps into creative processes serves as a catalyst for elevating humanity's collective productivity and overall well-being. Whether it's an artist seeking a muse or an organization striving to cultivate a culture of innovation, acknowledging the profound influence of a nap can be transformative. Embracing the myriad benefits of napping enables both individuals and businesses to tap into their creative reservoirs, thereby contributing to a future brimming with innovation and fulfillment.

Chapter 10. Napping for Energy Restoration

Today, where productivity is valued more than anything else, it's no wonder that many of us find ourselves feeling tired and drained. The constant demands of work, family, and social commitments can leave us feeling overwhelmed and depleted of energy. But what if there was a simple solution to restore our energy levels and enhance our overall well-being? Enter the power of napping.

Napping has long been regarded as a luxury or a sign of laziness, but recent scientific research has shown that it is a powerful tool for restoring energy and improving productivity. In fact, numerous studies have demonstrated the positive effects of napping on cognitive function, creativity, and mood. When we take a nap, we give our bodies and minds the opportunity to rest and recharge, allowing us to perform at our best.

One of the key benefits of napping is its ability to enhance our cognitive function. When we are sleep-deprived, our attention span, memory, and decision-making abilities suffer. However, a short nap of just 20–30 minutes has been shown to significantly improve these cognitive functions. By taking a nap during the day, we can reset our brains and improve our ability to focus and concentrate, leading to increased productivity and efficiency.

Napping also has a profound impact on our creativity. Research has shown that during sleep, our brains consolidate information and make connections between seemingly unrelated ideas. This means that when we wake up from a nap, we are more likely to have new insights and creative solutions to problems. So, instead of struggling to come up with fresh ideas, a short nap can provide the mental clarity and inspiration needed to think creatively.

Napping for Energy Restoration

Napping has been proven to boost our mood and overall well-being. When we are overtired, we are more likely to experience negative emotions such as irritability and stress. However, a nap can help regulate our emotions and reduce the risk of mood disorders. By giving ourselves permission to rest, we can improve our mental health and foster a positive outlook on life.

Napping is not a sign of laziness, but rather a powerful tool for enhancing our productivity and well-being. By taking a short nap during the day, we can restore our energy levels, improve our cognitive function and creativity, and boost our mood. So, let go of any guilt or stigma associated with napping and embrace its transformative effects. The power of a nap is within your reach – harness it and elevate your productivity and well-being.

Combating fatigue and preventing burnout with naps

Napping for Energy Restoration

It is no surprise that fatigue and burnout have become prevalent issues affecting individuals from all levels of society. The constant pressure to meet deadlines, juggle responsibilities, and maintain a work-life balance can take a toll on our physical and mental well-being. However, there is a simple yet powerful solution that can transform our productivity and overall well-being: the power of a nap.

Welcome to the subchapter on "Combating Fatigue and Preventing Burnout with Naps" from the book "Power Nap: Elevating Humanity's Productivity and Well-being." This chapter is addressed to all of humanity, as everyone can benefit from harnessing the power of naps to combat fatigue and prevent burnout.

Fatigue is a natural consequence of our bodies and minds working tirelessly, and it can negatively impact our performance, decision-making abilities, and overall quality of life. Burnout, on the other hand, is a state of chronic exhaustion that leaves us feeling emotionally drained and disengaged from our work and personal lives. The good news is that napping is a scientifically proven method to combat fatigue and prevent burnout.

Naps are not just for children or the lazy; they are a strategic tool that can enhance our productivity, creativity, and well-being. By taking a short nap, typically ranging from 15 to 30 minutes, we can recharge our batteries and rejuvenate our minds. Napping boosts our cognitive abilities, improves memory consolidation, enhances problem-solving skills, and increases our overall alertness and focus.

Moreover, naps have a profound impact on our emotional well-being. They help reduce stress, increase positive mood, and lower the risk of developing mental health issues such as anxiety and depression. Napping allows us to hit the reset button, giving us the opportunity to approach our tasks and challenges with a fresh perspective and renewed energy.

In a society that often glorifies overworking and sacrificing sleep, it is crucial to recognize the tremendous benefits of incorporating naps into our daily routines. By prioritizing self-care and embracing the power of a nap, we can prevent burnout, boost our productivity, and elevate our overall well-being.

So, humanity, it is time to reclaim our energy and embrace the transformative power of naps. Let us debunk the myths surrounding napping and embrace this natural and effective tool to combat fatigue and prevent burnout. By doing so, we can unlock our full potential, elevate our productivity, and enhance our overall quality of life. Remember, a well-rested individual is a thriving individual, and together, we can create a world that values the POWER of a nap.

Chapter 11. Napping as a sustainable energy source

Welcome to "Power Nap: Elevating Humanity's Productivity and Well-being." In this subchapter, we dive into the remarkable concept of napping as a sustainable energy source. We explore the POWER of a NAP and how it can revolutionize our lives and the world around us.

Napping has long been associated with laziness or unproductivity, but recent scientific research has unveiled its tremendous potential. As we delve deeper into the subject, we discover that napping holds the key to unlocking sustainable energy sources that can benefit both individuals and the planet.

The POWER of a NAP lies in its ability to rejuvenate and recharge our bodies and minds. When we nap, we tap into the natural rhythm of our circadian cycle, allowing us to restore depleted energy levels and enhance cognitive function. By embracing naps, we become more alert, creative, and efficient in our daily tasks.

But how can napping become a sustainable energy source? The answer lies in the concept of energy conservation. In a world grappling with the challenges of depleting resources and climate change, we need to explore alternative sources of energy – ones that are renewable and environmentally friendly. Surprisingly, napping holds the potential to fulfill this requirement.

Consider the idea of "nap pods" strategically placed in workplaces, public spaces, and even homes. These innovative sleep stations would harness the energy generated during napping and convert it into a usable form, such as electricity. As individuals rejuvenate themselves, they simultaneously contribute to the energy grid, reducing the reliance on conventional, non-renewable sources.

Napping as a sustainable energy source

Imagine a future where every nap taken helps power a city or a village, where energy sustainability is no longer a distant dream but a reality. This vision can be achieved through the collective efforts of humanity, recognizing the POWER of a NAP and its potential to revolutionize our energy consumption patterns.

Additionally, napping as a sustainable energy source can have a profound impact on our well-being. As we prioritize rest and rejuvenation, we reduce stress levels, improve mental health, and enhance overall productivity. This positive cycle of well-being contributes to a happier and healthier society.

Napping as a sustainable energy source holds immense promise for the future of humanity. By embracing the POWER of a NAP, we can tap into renewable sources of energy, reduce our carbon footprint, and improve our well-being. Let us strive towards a future where napping is valued for its restorative benefits and celebrated as a catalyst for positive change.

Napping as a sustainable energy source

Maximizing productivity through strategic napping

Welcome to the subchapter on "Maximizing productivity through strategic napping" from the book "Power Nap: Elevating Humanity's Productivity and Well-being." In this chapter, we will explore the incredible power of a nap and how it can transform your productivity levels. Whether you are a student, a working professional, or anyone seeking to enhance their well-being, this chapter is for you.

Napping has long been regarded as a sign of laziness or unproductiveness. However, recent scientific research has debunked this misconception, revealing the unbelievable benefits of strategic napping. Naps can boost cognitive function, improve memory retention, enhance creativity, and increase overall productivity.

1. Cognitive Enhancement: Strategic napping has been shown to significantly improve

cognitive abilities. A short power nap can help recharge your brain, improve focus, and enhance problem-solving skills. By taking a break and allowing your mind to rest, you can return to your tasks with a refreshed mental state, leading to increased productivity.

2. Memory Consolidation: Napping plays a crucial role in memory consolidation. During sleep, the brain processes and stores information, enhancing memory retention. By incorporating a nap into your daily routine, you can optimize your learning and retain information more effectively, ultimately boosting your productivity.

3. Creativity Boost: Napping can also stimulate creative thinking. Studies have shown that during a nap, the brain engages in unique neural processes that help foster creativity. By capitalizing on this opportunity, you can tap

into your creative potential, leading to innovative solutions and improved productivity.

Chapter 12. Implementing Strategic Napping:

To maximize the benefits of napping, it is important to adopt a strategic approach. Here are some tips to help you integrate napping into your routine effectively:

a. Timing: Napping for too long or too close to bedtime can disrupt your sleep schedule. Aim for short power naps, ideally around 15–30 minutes, to avoid feeling groggy upon waking.

b. Environment: Create a comfortable and quiet environment conducive to sleep. Find a peaceful spot where you can relax and recharge without distractions.

c. Consistency: Establish a regular napping routine to allow your body and mind to adapt. Consistency is key to reaping the maximum benefits of strategic napping.

Implementing Strategic Napping:

Conclusion: Incorporating strategic napping into your daily routine can revolutionize your productivity levels. Embrace the power of a nap, unleash your creativity, improve cognitive function, and enhance memory retention. By understanding and harnessing the potential of napping, you can elevate both your productivity and overall well-being.

The Effect of Napping on Well-being

Today, stress has become an inevitable part of our lives. With hectic schedules, demanding jobs, and constant connectivity, it's no wonder that stress levels have skyrocketed. But what if there was a simple and effective way to combat stress and boost our overall well-being? Enter the power of napping.

Napping, often underestimated and overlooked, has remarkable stress-reducing abilities. In fact, research has shown that a well-timed nap can do wonders for our mental and physical health. It provides a much-needed break from the daily

Implementing Strategic Napping:

grind, allowing our minds and bodies to recharge and rejuvenate.

One of the significant benefits of napping is its ability to reduce cortisol levels, which is a hormone released in response to stress. When we are constantly under pressure, our bodies produce excessive amounts of cortisol, leading to a range of negative effects on our health, including increased anxiety, decreased immune function, and even weight gain. However, a power nap can help counteract these harmful effects by lowering cortisol levels and promoting relaxation.

Moreover, napping has been shown to enhance cognitive function and improve memory and learning abilities. When we are stressed, our minds become cluttered, making it difficult to focus and retain information. By taking a brief nap, we allow our brains to consolidate and process the information we have absorbed throughout the day. This results in improved cognitive performance and increased productivity once we wake up.

Implementing Strategic Napping:

Napping also plays a crucial role in boosting our mood and overall well-being. It provides a temporary escape from the stressors of life, allowing us to reset and approach challenges with a fresh perspective. A nap acts as a reset button for our emotions, helping to alleviate feelings of irritability, frustration, and anxiety. By taking a nap, we give ourselves the opportunity to recharge emotionally, leading to a more positive and balanced outlook.

Incorporating napping into our daily routines may seem like a luxury, but it is a powerful tool for stress reduction and overall well-being. By recognizing the importance of self-care and giving ourselves permission to take a break, we can harness the immense benefits of napping. So, the next time you feel overwhelmed or stressed, remember the Power Nap and give yourself the gift of a rejuvenating nap. Your mind, body, and overall productivity will thank you.

Napping as a stress management technique

Implementing Strategic Napping:

Stress has become an inevitable part of our lives. The constant pressure to perform, meet deadlines, and juggle multiple responsibilities can take a toll on our mental and physical well-being. Fortunately, there is a simple yet effective solution that can help alleviate stress and restore our energy levels: napping.

Napping, often underrated and overlooked, has been proven to be a powerful stress management technique. Research has shown that a short nap of just 20–30 minutes can have remarkable benefits for our overall health and well-being. It provides a much-needed break from the daily grind, allowing our minds and bodies to recharge and rejuvenate.

One of the key advantages of napping as a stress management technique is its ability to reduce the production of stress hormones such as cortisol. When we are stressed, our bodies release cortisol, which can lead to a range of negative effects, including sleep disturbances, anxiety, and mood swings. By taking a nap, we

Implementing Strategic Napping:

can significantly lower cortisol levels, promoting a sense of calmness and relaxation.

Moreover, napping enhances our cognitive function and improves mental clarity. When we are stressed, our ability to concentrate and make decisions diminishes. However, a nap can help restore these faculties, allowing us to think more clearly and tackle challenges with a renewed perspective. Additionally, napping has been linked to improved memory consolidation, helping us retain information and learn more effectively.

Beyond the cognitive benefits, napping offers a physical reprieve from stress. It reduces muscle tension, alleviates headaches, and lowers blood pressure. By giving our bodies, a chance to rest and recover, napping contributes to our overall physical well-being, reducing the risk of stress-related ailments such as heart disease and obesity.

Furthermore, napping can enhance our mood and emotional resilience. It provides an

Implementing Strategic Napping:

opportunity to escape from the pressures of everyday life and find solace in a moment of tranquility. This, in turn, can lead to increased happiness, reduced irritability, and improved emotional stability.

Incorporating napping as a regular part of our routine can have a transformative effect on our productivity and well-being. By recognizing the power of a nap, we can unlock the potential to elevate our performance, creativity, and overall quality of life. So, let us embrace Power Nap and make it an essential tool in our stress management toolbox, for the betterment of humanity.

Chapter 13. The Role of Napping in Regulating Cortisol Levels

The human body follows natural circadian rhythms that regulate hormone production over a 24-hour period. One key hormone impacted by these daily cycles is cortisol. Secreted by the adrenal glands, cortisol is known as the "stress hormone" due to its mobilizing effects. Cortisol levels tend to peak in the early morning then decline throughout the day, reaching their lowest point around midnight. This daily fluctuation assists proper bodily functioning. However, chronic stress can disrupt healthy cortisol rhythms, leading to elevated evening cortisol which can impair sleep, metabolism, and immunity. Fortunately, napping has been shown to help regulate cortisol secretion to healthier patterns.

The Role of Napping in Regulating Cortisol Levels

Studies Demonstrate Napping Lowers Cortisol

Multiple studies have now clearly demonstrated that daytime napping lowers cortisol secretions and reduces stress arousal in the body and mind. One study published in the Endocrine Society's Journal of Clinical Endocrinology & Metabolism found that levels of cortisol significantly decreased after participants took a 60–90-minute naps in the afternoon. Additionally, growth hormone levels increased during napping, which aids stress recovery. The researchers concluded that afternoon napping has beneficial impacts on hormone regulation that helps counteract the negative effects of stress.

Further evidence of napping's cortisol-lowering powers comes from a study conducted by University of California, Berkeley researchers. In a controlled crossover study, participants both took a 60-minute midday nap and engaged in an equal period of quiet rest without sleep. Cortisol levels decreased during both nap and rest conditions, but the decline was more than twice as great during the nap. Napping had a stronger normalizing effect on cortisol than just resting quietly without sleep. The researchers theorized that the initial boosted cortisol from lying down may have allowed for a greater subsequent reduction during napping. The findings provide confirmation that daytime naps can effectively reduce cortisol levels.

Optimized timing is key

While napping clearly lowers cortisol, the timing of when you nap makes a significant difference. Cortisol levels naturally rise from when we wake up in the morning until peaking around midday. Then levels steadily decline throughout the afternoon and reach a daily nadir around midnight before the cycle repeats. If you take a nap too late in the day, close to bedtime, it can interfere with this natural rhythm and healthy overnight cortisol decrease.

A study published in the journal Psych neuroendocrinology examined the impact of nap timing on cortisol levels. Participants were either permitted a 30-minute nap before 3pm or prohibited from napping. The study found that those who napped before 3pm showed significantly greater reductions in cortisol later in the day compared to non-nappers. However, when participants napped after 3pm, their cortisol did not decrease as expected in the evening. This demonstrates the importance of taking a nap earlier in the day, ideally between 1-3pm, to aid healthy cortisol regulation.

Chapter 14. Light Napping of 20–30 Minutes Ideal

In addition to proper timing, the ideal nap duration for lowering cortisol appears to be a shorter 20–30-minute nap. Research published in the journal Sleep examined cortisol levels after varying nap lengths. The results showed that just a 30-minute nap was sufficient to significantly reduce cortisol versus no nap. However, longer naps of 60 minutes produced less of a cortisol-lowering effect. A short 20–30-minute nap may avoid deleterious cortisol spikes upon awakening from longer naps. Short power naps deliver the benefits without the drawbacks.

Napping may influence cortisol levels through impacts on stress-response regions of the brain. Neuroimaging studies have demonstrated that midday naps can reduce activity in the amygdala and other areas associated with stress and negative emotions. Turning down activation in these areas through napping then signals the adrenal glands to secrete less cortisol. This brain-adrenal axis is one mechanism by which naps may exert regulatory effects on cortisol production.

Regular Napping Habit Key for Lasting Impact

The body adapts to patterns and consistent habits. Research has shown that the benefits of napping are amplified when it becomes a stable routine versus random occurrence. Adults with regular napping habits have been found to have greater overnight drops in cortisol compared to non-habitual nappers. The advantages of napping become more pronounced over time as the body's systems adjust to the restorative periods. Establishing a daily 20–30-minute nap can result in positive cortisol regulation.

One study allowed participants two 20-minute practice naps in the lab, which established an initial napping habit. These participants were then asked to continue daily nap practice at home. Over the three-week home napping period, the habitual nappers experienced significant incremental reductions in evening cortisol levels compared to a control group. This demonstrates the cortisol-regulating power of consistent daily napping.

Societal Acceptance of Napping Still Needed

While adoption of workplace napping policies has slowly increased in recent years, there is still progress needed toward broader social acceptance of napping's benefits. Millions of years of evolution support an afternoon nap as a natural circadian rhythm, yet the stigma remains. Education on the extensive research-backed advantages of napping for productivity, health, learning, and stress should continue. Normalization by leading companies and public figures openly embracing daily napping habits can help drive cultural change.

Given the alarming rise in stress and burnout, promoting napping as an accessible and

Light Napping of 20–30 Minutes Ideal

effective self-care tool is prudent. Companies investing in employee nap rooms and designated nap times will be rewarded with a happier, healthier and higher-performing workforce. We owe it to ourselves and future generations to overcome outdated assumptions and acknowledge the positive impacts of strategic napping. Only once napping is woven back into the fabric of everyday life and culture can we fully harness its untapped potential.

The Napping Solution:

Napping has long been known to provide a quick recharge, but its impact goes far beyond just feeling refreshed. Research has shown that napping can play a crucial role in regulating cortisol levels, effectively reducing stress and improving our overall mental and physical health.

When we nap, our bodies enter a state of relaxation, allowing cortisol levels to decrease. This reduction in cortisol helps us feel more relaxed and enables us to think more clearly,

Light Napping of 20–30 Minutes Ideal

make better decisions, and boost our productivity. By incorporating regular napping into our daily routine, we can create a buffer against stress and enhance our ability to handle challenging situations with composure and clarity.

Chapter 15. Napping Techniques:

To fully benefit from the cortisol-regulating effects of napping, it is important to understand the best practices for effective napping. Short power naps of 20–30 minutes have been found to be the most effective in reducing cortisol levels and improving alertness. These power naps can be taken at any time of the day, depending on individual preferences and schedules.

Creating a Nap-Friendly Environment:

To optimize the benefits of napping, it is essential to create a nap-friendly environment. Find a quiet and comfortable space where you can relax without interruptions. Dim the lights, use soft music or white noise to drown out external distractions, and consider using a cozy blanket or eye mask to enhance relaxation. By designing a

Napping Techniques:

soothing environment, you can maximize the cortisol-regulating benefits of your nap.

Understanding the role of napping in regulating cortisol levels is a crucial step towards harnessing the power of a nap. By incorporating regular napping into our daily routine, we can effectively manage stress, improve cognitive function, and elevate our overall well-being. Embrace the Power Nap and unlock your true potential for productivity and happiness.

Napping for emotional well-being

In this fast-paced and demanding world, it's easy to feel overwhelmed and emotionally drained. We often find ourselves grappling with stress, anxiety, and a constant need to be productive. But what if there was a simple yet powerful solution to boost our emotional well-being and regain control over our emotions? Enter the incredible power of napping.

Napping has long been associated with physical rejuvenation and increased alertness, but its benefits extend far beyond that. Research has

Napping Techniques:

shown that napping can have a profound impact on our emotional state, helping us manage stress, regulate our emotions, and enhance our overall well-being.

One of the keyways napping supports emotional well-being is by reducing the effects of stress. When we nap, our bodies enter a state of relaxation, allowing our minds to unwind and release the built-up tension. This not only helps us feel calmer and more at ease but also restores our emotional equilibrium. By taking a short nap during a stressful day, we give ourselves the opportunity to recharge and face challenges with a renewed sense of emotional resilience.

Moreover, napping plays a crucial role in emotional regulation. When we lack sufficient sleep, our emotions can become more volatile and harder to manage. However, a well-timed nap can help stabilize our mood and improve emotional control. It gives our brain the chance to process and integrate experiences, promoting emotional clarity and a more balanced outlook. By incorporating regular naps into our routine,

Napping Techniques:

we can better navigate the difficulties of life, fostering emotional stability and well-being.

Additionally, napping enhances our ability to manage and cope with negative emotions. When we're sleep-deprived or emotionally exhausted, even minor setbacks can feel overwhelming. However, a nap can reset our emotional state, enabling us to approach challenges with a fresh perspective and increased resilience. It allows us to distance ourselves from negative emotions, allowing us the space to reframe our thoughts and find healthier ways to cope.

Napping is not just a tool for physical rest; it is a powerful means to boost our emotional well-being. By incorporating napping into our daily lives, we can effectively manage stress, regulate our emotions, and strengthen our overall resilience. The transformative effects of napping on our emotional state have the potential to elevate humanity's productivity and well-being. So, let us embrace the power of a nap and unlock the full potential of our emotional health.

Napping Techniques:

Napping for Memory Enhancement

In our fast-paced world, finding effective methods to enhance memory and cognitive functions has become a paramount concern for many individuals. Surprisingly, one of the most powerful tools at our disposal is also one of the most overlooked – napping. Yes, that rejuvenating afternoon siesta may hold the key to unlocking your brain's full potential and boosting memory.

Napping has long been associated with rest and relaxation, but recent scientific studies have shed light on its remarkable benefits for memory enhancement. When we sleep, our brain undergoes a process called memory consolidation, where it strengthens and solidifies newly acquired information. Napping serves as an intermediary between short-term and long-term memory, helping to transfer information from one to the other more efficiently.

Research has shown that even short power naps of 20-30 minutes can significantly improve

Napping Techniques:

memory and cognitive performance. During this brief period, our brain enters a state of light sleep known as stage 2, which is ideal for memory consolidation. As a result, napping enhances our ability to remember facts, learn new skills, and retain information for longer periods.

Furthermore, napping has been found to boost creativity and problem-solving abilities. During sleep, our brain is free from distractions, allowing it to make new connections and associations between different pieces of information. This unique cognitive process, facilitated by napping, promotes innovative thinking and enhances our ability to find creative solutions to complex problems.

The benefits of napping extend beyond memory enhancement. Research has shown that regular napping can also improve overall well-being and productivity. By giving our brain, a chance to rest and recharge, napping helps combat fatigue and reduces stress levels. This, in turn, leads to increased focus, heightened alertness,

Napping Techniques:

and improved mood – all essential factors for optimal productivity and well-being.

Napping is a powerful tool that can significantly enhance memory, cognitive abilities, and overall productivity. By incorporating short power naps into our daily routine, we can tap into the full potential of our brains and elevate our performance in various aspects of life. So, embrace the power of a nap and unlock the hidden potential within you. Your memory, creativity, and well-being will thank you for it.

Chapter 16. How napping improves memory consolidation

In our fast-paced world, the concept of napping is often associated with laziness or unproductivity. However, scientific research has revealed that taking a nap can enhance memory consolidation, leading to improved cognitive abilities and overall productivity. In this subchapter, we will explore the fascinating connection between napping and memory, shedding light on the powerful effects of a well-timed nap.

Memory consolidation is the process by which our brains convert short-term memories into long-term memories. It is during this crucial phase that information becomes integrated into our existing knowledge, enhancing our ability to recall and apply it later. Numerous studies have shown that napping plays a vital role in

How napping improves memory consolidation

facilitating this consolidation process, leading to better retention and retrieval of information.

One of the key mechanisms through which napping improves memory consolidation is by allowing our brains to rest and recharge. When we engage in mental activities throughout the day, our brains accumulate fatigue and become less efficient at processing and storing information. By taking a nap, we provide our brains with the opportunity to rejuvenate, allowing them to better encode and consolidate memories.

Napping has been found to enhance the activation of the hippocampus; a brain region crucial for memory formation. During sleep, the hippocampus replays and strengthens the neural connections associated with recently acquired information, solidifying memories. By incorporating a nap into our daily routine, we can optimize this process, leading to more robust memories and improved learning abilities.

How napping improves memory consolidation

Interestingly, the duration and timing of a nap also play a significant role in memory consolidation. Research suggests that short power naps, ranging from 10 to 30 minutes, are particularly effective in enhancing memory without causing grogginess upon waking. Additionally, napping in the mid-afternoon, when our natural circadian rhythm prompts a dip in alertness, maximizes the benefits of memory consolidation.

Napping is not merely a luxury or a sign of idleness; it is a powerful tool that enhances memory consolidation and boosts overall productivity. By understanding the science behind this phenomenon, we can harness the Power Nap to elevate our cognitive abilities and well-being. So, let us embrace the POWER of a NAP and unlock the full potential of our minds.

Napping techniques to enhance learning and retention

Finding time to rest and recharge has become increasingly difficult. However, science has

How napping improves memory consolidation

shown us that taking a nap during the day can have tremendous benefits for our overall well-being and productivity. In this subchapter, we will explore various napping techniques that can enhance learning and retention, giving you the POWER of a NAP.

1. The Power Nap: This technique involves taking a short nap of around 20 minutes. Research has shown that this duration can help improve alertness, concentration, and cognitive performance. By allowing your brain to rest and reset, you can enhance your ability to learn and retain information.

2. The Memory Boost: If you're looking to retain and consolidate current information, try the Memory Boost technique. Start by reviewing the material before taking a nap. During your nap, your brain will process and organize the information, leading to better retention. Upon waking, review the material again, reinforcing what you have learned.

3. The Creative Nap: Napping can also boost creativity and problem-solving abilities. To tap into your creative potential, try taking a nap after brainstorming or working on a challenging task. During sleep, your brain continues to work on problems in the background, making connections and generating innovative ideas. Upon waking, you might find yourself approaching the task with fresh perspectives and innovative solutions.

4. The Learning Break: If you're engaged in a long study session, taking regular napping breaks can help optimize your learning. Instead of powering through for hours on end, try breaking your study time into shorter intervals, punctuated by naps. This technique, known as the Pomodoro Technique, has been shown to improve focus, concentration, and information retention.

5. Nap Meditation: Napping can also be a powerful tool for relaxation and stress reduction. By combining napping with meditation techniques, you can create a deeply restorative

experience. Find a quiet and comfortable space, set a timer for 20-30 minutes, and engage in mindful breathing or visualization exercises. This technique can help calm your mind, reduce anxiety, and enhance overall well-being.

Remember, the key to successful napping is to find what works best for you. Experiment with different techniques and durations to discover the nap routine that enhances your learning and retention abilities. By harnessing the POWER of a NAP, you can elevate your productivity, creativity, and overall well-being, leading to a more fulfilled and successful life.

Napping for academic and professional success

Today, the demands of academia and the professional sphere often leave us feeling overwhelmed and exhausted. However, what if we told you that there is a simple and effective solution to enhance your productivity and well-being? It's time to unlock the power of napping.

Napping has long been associated with laziness or a lack of ambition, but recent scientific research has proven otherwise. In fact, napping has been shown to have numerous cognitive and health benefits, making it a valuable tool for academic and professional success.

One of the most significant advantages of napping is its ability to improve memory and enhance learning. When we nap, our brains consolidate information, allowing us to better retain and recall what we have learned. This means that by incorporating a short nap into your study or work routine, you can boost your ability to absorb current information and improve overall performance.

Furthermore, napping has a profound impact on our creativity and problem-solving skills. During sleep, our brains engage in a process called memory reactivation, where they form new connections and find innovative solutions to complex problems. By taking a nap, you give your brain the opportunity to tap into its creative potential, enabling you to approach challenges with fresh perspectives and find unique solutions.

How napping improves memory consolidation

But napping isn't just beneficial for intellectual pursuits; it also has a significant impact on our emotional well-being. When we are sleep-deprived, our mood and overall mental health suffer. However, a nap can help reset our emotional state, alleviating stress, anxiety, and even depression. By prioritizing rest and rejuvenation, you can enhance your emotional resilience and maintain a positive outlook, even in the face of demanding academic or professional pressures.

Incorporating napping into your daily routine doesn't require hours of sleep or disrupt your schedule. Even a short power nap of 20-30 minutes can work wonders. Find a quiet and comfortable space, set an alarm, and allow yourself to unwind and recharge. You'll be amazed at the transformation it can bring to your academic and professional life.

Summary, don't underestimate the power of a nap. By embracing this simple yet effective practice, you can enhance your cognitive abilities, unleash your creative potential, and improve your emotional well-being. So, let go of the misconceptions and embrace Power Nap – a tool that elevates humanity's productivity and well-being.

Chapter 17. The Healing Power of Naps:

Continually pushing our bodies without pause can lead to impaired immune function, increased inflammation, weight gain, and lowered physical health. Emerging research demonstrates that brief daytime napping offers a simple yet powerful antidote. Beyond just mental recovery, napping provides profound physiological benefits by boosting immunity, aiding healing, regulating key hormones, lowering blood pressure, and promoting overall physical wellness.

Napping to Support Immune Function

Sleep plays an integral role in proper immune system functioning. During sleep, our bodies produce infection-fighting antibodies and immune cells called cytokines. However, chronic partial sleep deprivation impairs this restorative immune process. Getting insufficient sleep leaves us more prone to illness. Luckily, catching up on sleep through napping can reverse the immune-suppressing effects of sleep loss.

Studies have found that people who take short regular naps have higher levels of lymphocytes compared with non-nappers, boosting resistance to disease. Research also shows that napping triggers a burst of cytokine production, enhancing anti-inflammatory responses. In one Stanford University study, volunteers were given vaccines. Those who napped after the injection produced more antibodies in response compared to those who stayed awake, demonstrating improved immune memory from the naps. The researchers concluded that napping supports our ability to fight foreign pathogens.

Accelerating Physical Recovery and Healing

Beyond strengthening immunity, research confirms sleep facilitates cellular repair and recovery from injury or illness. During sleep, our bodies release key hormones involved in tissue healing and muscle growth. Deep non-REM sleep is especially restorative. After daytime physical exertion, napping provides an opportunity for this restorative slow-wave sleep to enhance the body's natural healing abilities.

Studies have shown improved athletic performance and accelerated muscle repair in athletes who nap regularly. Research published in the Journal of Strength and Conditioning found that college basketball players who napped for at least 2 hours per day had less occurrence of injury. Their bodies had time to fully regenerate muscle tissue between practices. For anyone facing surgery, illness or injury, sufficient restorative sleep is crucial. Daytime napping can assist the healing process when nighttime sleep is disrupted.

Regulating Metabolism and Appetite

Beyond directly facilitating tissue repair, napping influences metabolism and weight control through impacts on hormone levels. Two key players here are growth hormone and cortisol. Growth hormones are produced during slow-wave sleep and help increase muscle mass and burn fat. Cortisol is the stress hormone that signals hunger cravings when elevated. Studies confirm that daytime napping boosts growth hormone secretion while reducing cortisol levels, optimizing metabolism.

Researchers have found that people who habitually nap have higher growth hormone levels and lower BMIs compared to non-nappers. Another study published in the Journal of Clinical Endocrinology & Metabolism demonstrated that participants who took a 1-hour nap in the afternoon experienced a 5-fold increase in growth hormone secretion. The researchers concluded daytime napping helps regulate hormones that influence obesity risk. By napping, we tap into physiological pathways that enhance weight control and reduce overeating urges.

Lowering Blood Pressure

The Healing Power of Naps: How Napping Promotes Physical Health

Given its stress-reducing effects, it's logical that napping may also lower blood pressure. High blood pressure significantly increases risks for stroke, heart attack and cardiovascular disease. However, brief midday naps have been shown to help lower BP into healthy ranges, particularly for individuals already diagnosed with hypertension.

In a Greek research study, participants with high BP were split into two groups: a nap group who slept for 30 minutes at midday and a control group who stayed awake reading. At the end of the 8-week study period, the napping group showed significant reductions in 24-hour BP averages compared to controls. The researchers concluded that midday napping can be an effective intervention for hypertension. Other studies have also observed decreased BP after napping compared to not napping. Daytime sleep allows cardiovascular restoration.

Optimizing Nap Habits for Health

The Healing Power of Naps: How Napping Promotes Physical Health

As with any healthy habit, consistency and timing are key to reaping maximum benefits. Taking a daily nap at the same time each day allows your body's rhythms to align to best utilize the rest. The early to mid-afternoon (1-3pm) tends to be the ideal nap window, when nature dips in alertness and slower brain waves prime us for deeper sleep. Limiting nap length to approximately 20-30 minutes prevents you from entering the deeper sleep stages, allowing you to wake up feeling refreshed.

Make sure your napping environment is cool, quiet, and dark. Use eye masks, ear plugs or sleep headphones with white noise to set the stage for quality rest. To further boost your nap's restorative effects, pair it with other lifestyle measures like regular exercise, a healthy diet, and stress management techniques. By sticking with your routine over the long term, napping becomes an easy self-care habit with compounded health benefits.

The Bottom Line

The Healing Power of Naps: How Napping Promotes Physical Health

Emerging research points out that napping is far more than just a luxury: it is a science-backed strategy for optimizing physical wellness. The unique physiological benefits of brief daytime sleep on immunity, healing, hormones, and heart health make the nap a powerful yet accessible tool for improving health. In our productivity-obsessed culture, granting yourself permission to nap may require a perspective shift. However, the long-term dividends for your overall wellbeing make an afternoon nap more than worth that investment. Our bodies are hardwired for cycles of activity and rest. Let's embrace the gift of the nap and reclaim this ancestral pathway to health.

Chapter 18. Napping's impact on cardiovascular health

In the fast-paced world we live in, finding time to rest and rejuvenate can be a challenge. However, incorporating a short nap into your daily routine can have a significant impact on your cardiovascular health. In this subchapter, we will explore the powerful effects of napping and how it can contribute to elevating humanity's productivity and well-being.

Numerous studies have shown that regular napping can lower the risk of cardiovascular diseases such as heart attacks and strokes. During a nap, our bodies enter a state of relaxation, allowing our blood pressure and heart rate to decrease. This reduction in stress on the cardiovascular system promotes better overall heart health.

Furthermore, napping has been proven to improve the function of blood vessels, leading to better blood flow and circulation. This is particularly important for those at risk of developing cardiovascular problems. By taking a short nap, individuals can enhance their body's ability to deliver oxygen and nutrients to vital organs, reducing the strain on the heart and preventing the onset of cardiovascular diseases.

Additionally, napping has been found to regulate hormone levels, particularly cortisol, which is responsible for managing stress. Elevated levels of cortisol can contribute to increased blood pressure and inflammation, both of which are risk factors for heart disease. By incorporating a nap into your daily routine, you can effectively reduce cortisol levels, promoting a healthier cardiovascular system.

The benefits of napping are not limited to the cardiovascular system alone. Taking a short nap can also improve cognitive function, memory retention, and overall mood. By boosting productivity and well-being, napping allows

Napping's impact on cardiovascular health

individuals to approach their work and personal life with a renewed sense of energy and focus.

The impact of napping on cardiovascular health cannot be underestimated. By incorporating a short nap into your daily routine, you can lower your risk of developing heart diseases, improve blood flow, regulate hormone levels, and enhance overall well-being. The power of a nap lies not only in its ability to provide rest, but also in its ability to elevate humanity's productivity and well-being. Embrace the Power Nap and unlock the potential for a healthier and more fulfilling life.

Napping for immune system support

Today, it appears that everyone is constantly on the go, juggling multiple responsibilities and facing important levels of stress. With our attention divided among work, family, and personal commitments, it is no wonder that our immune systems often take a hit. But what if there was a simple and effective way to boost your immune system? Enter the power of a nap.

Napping's impact on cardiovascular health

In this subchapter, we will explore the astonishing benefits of napping for immune system support and how it can significantly elevate your productivity and well-being. Napping has long been associated with relaxation and rejuvenation, but recent scientific research has revealed its profound impact on our immune health.

When we are sleep-deprived or experiencing chronic stress, our immune system weakens, making us more susceptible to illnesses and infections. However, taking a nap can help counteract these effects by enhancing our body's natural defense mechanisms. During sleep, our immune system releases proteins called cytokines that help promote sleep and fight off infections. Napping allows our body to produce an optimal amount of these cytokines, thereby strengthening our immune system.

Napping has been shown to reduce the production of cortisol, the stress hormone responsible for suppressing immune function. By taking a short nap, you can give your body a

Napping's impact on cardiovascular health

chance to reset, lower cortisol levels, and restore balance to your immune system.

The benefits of napping go beyond immune support. Research has also shown that regular napping can improve cognitive function, memory retention, and creativity. By allowing your brain to rest and recharge, you can enhance your overall productivity and mental well-being.

To harness the power of a nap for immune system support, it is essential to follow a few guidelines. Aim for a nap duration of around 20-30 minutes, as this is the optimal length to reap the benefits without entering deep sleep. Find a quiet and comfortable space, free from distractions, where you can relax and unwind. Set an alarm to ensure you don't oversleep and disrupt your nighttime rest.

Summary, napping is a simple yet powerful tool to support your immune system and elevate your overall well-being. By incorporating short naps into your daily routine, you can enhance your body's natural defense mechanisms, reduce stress, and boost productivity. So, embrace the Power Nap and take a step towards a healthier and more productive life.

Napping as a tool for weight management

Today, weight management has become a pressing concern for many individuals. The struggle to maintain a healthy weight has led to the rise of various diet plans and exercise regimes. However, there is one powerful tool that often goes unnoticed in the quest for weight management – napping.

Napping has long been associated with relaxation and rejuvenation, but its benefits extend far beyond just feeling rested. Research has shown that napping can play a significant role in weight management by positively impacting our metabolism, appetite, and overall well-being.

One of the keyways in which napping aids weight management is by boosting metabolism. When we nap, our body's metabolic rate increases, helping us burn calories more efficiently. Studies have found that a short nap of 20-30 minutes can increase metabolic activity by up to 20%, which can have a significant impact on weight loss or maintenance.

Moreover, napping can also help regulate appetite and cravings. Lack of sleep has been linked to an increase in hunger hormones, leading to overeating and unhealthy food choices. By incorporating regular napping into our routine, we can address this issue. Napping helps balance the hormones responsible for appetite control, reducing cravings for high-calorie foods and promoting better portion control.

Beyond its direct effects on metabolism and appetite, napping also plays a crucial role in overall well-being. When we are well-rested, we are more likely to make healthier choices throughout the day. Napping enhances cognitive function, alertness, and decision-making abilities, making it easier for us to resist temptation and stick to our weight management goals.

Furthermore, napping has a positive impact on our stress levels. Chronic stress has been linked to weight gain and difficulty in losing weight. Napping is a natural stress reliever, promoting relaxation and reducing cortisol levels, which in turn helps control our weight.

Incorporating napping as a tool for weight management requires a strategic approach. It is essential to find the ideal time and duration for naps, ensuring they do not interfere with nighttime sleep. Short power naps during the mid-afternoon slump or after a heavy meal can be highly effective in reaping the benefits of napping for weight management.

Napping offers a powerful yet often overlooked tool for weight management. By boosting metabolism, regulating appetite, reducing stress, and enhancing overall well-being, napping can significantly contribute to achieving and maintaining a healthy weight. So, let us embrace the power of a nap and harness its potential to elevate humanity's productivity and well-being.

Chapter 19. Napping as a Lifestyle Choice

Napping, an age-old practice that has been embraced by numerous cultures throughout history, continues to face unnecessary societal stigma Today. In the subchapter "Overcoming Societal Stigma Surrounding Napping" of the book "Power Nap: Elevating Humanity's Productivity and Well-being," we delve into the misconceptions surrounding napping and explore the power it holds in enhancing our productivity and overall well-being.

In a society that glorifies busyness and labels napping as a sign of laziness or weakness, it is time we challenge these beliefs and reclaim the POWER of a NAP. Napping is not a form of idleness; instead, it is a strategic tool that can rejuvenate our minds, boost creativity, and increase our overall productivity.

Napping as a Lifestyle Choice

One of the primary reasons why napping faces societal stigma is the misconception that it is a waste of time. However, research has shown that a short nap can significantly improve cognitive function, memory retention, and information processing. By taking a nap, we recharge our brains, allowing us to approach tasks with renewed focus and clarity. It is through napping that we can tap into the hidden potential of our minds and unlock innovative solutions to complex problems.

Another misconception surrounding napping is its association with laziness. The truth is napping is not a sign of laziness but rather a sign of self-care and self-awareness. In today's hyper-connected world, where we are constantly bombarded with information and demands, taking a nap is an act of prioritizing our well-being. By allowing ourselves to rest and recharge, we can prevent burnout and maintain a healthy work-life balance.

Moreover, the stigma around napping is often fueled by a lack of understanding about sleep cycles and the benefits of power naps. Research has shown that a well-timed power nap can provide a significant energy boost, enhance alertness, and improve mood. By educating ourselves and others about the science behind napping, we can dispel the myths and misconceptions that prevent us from embracing this powerful tool.

Summary, it is time we challenge the societal stigma surrounding napping and embrace the POWER of a NAP. By recognizing the benefits of napping on our productivity, creativity, and overall well-being, we can elevate humanity's potential. Let us break free from the chains of societal expectations and reclaim our right to rest and rejuvenate. Embrace the Power Nap and unlock the extraordinary within you.

The cultural perception of napping

The cultural perception of napping is a fascinating subject that reveals a lot about the values and beliefs of different societies throughout history. In the book "Power Nap:

Napping as a Lifestyle Choice

Elevating Humanity's Productivity and Well-being," we explore how the perception of napping varies across cultures and its impact on productivity and well-being.

In many Western societies, napping has often been associated with laziness or lack of ambition. The prevailing cultural narrative promotes the idea that success and productivity require constant activity and working long hours without rest. However, this perspective is gradually changing as scientific research and anecdotal evidence demonstrate the numerous benefits of napping.

In contrast, several Eastern cultures have a long-standing tradition of embracing napping to recharge and improve mental focus. Countries like China, Japan, and Spain have a cultural acceptance of afternoon siestas, recognizing their positive impact on the overall well-being and productivity of individuals.

The cultural perception of napping also intersects with societal norms and workplace policies. In some countries, such as France, companies have implemented policies that allow employees to take a short nap during working hours. This progressive approach acknowledges the importance of rest and acknowledges that a well-rested employee is likely to be more productive and efficient.

Understanding the cultural perception of napping is essential for individuals and organizations seeking to optimize productivity and well-being. By challenging the negative stereotypes surrounding napping, we can create a cultural shift that recognizes the value of rest and rejuvenation.

Moreover, the power of a nap goes beyond mere rest. Research has shown that napping can improve cognitive function, memory retention, and creativity. It can also reduce stress, boost mood, and enhance overall mental and physical well-being.

As we delve deeper into the cultural perception of napping, it becomes evident that our attitudes towards rest and rejuvenation shape our daily lives and overall productivity. By embracing the positive aspects of napping and challenging cultural biases, we can unlock the full potential of the human mind and elevate our collective productivity and well-being.

"Power Nap: Elevating Humanity's Productivity and Well-being" aims to explore the cultural perception of napping, challenge societal norms, and provide evidence-based insights on the power of napping. By sharing stories, research, and practical tips, this subchapter seeks to empower humanity to harness the benefits of napping and revolutionize our approach to productivity and well-being.

Shifting societal attitudes towards napping

Recently, there has been a remarkable shift in societal attitudes towards napping. What was once seen as a sign of laziness or unproductivity is now being embraced as a powerful tool for enhancing productivity and overall well-being. This shift can be attributed to several factors, including scientific research, changing work cultures, and a growing understanding of the importance of self-care.

Scientific studies have played a significant role in changing societal perceptions about napping. Research has shown repeatedly that a well-timed nap can significantly improve cognitive function, memory retention, and creativity. Moreover, napping has been linked to reducing stress, boosting mood, and enhancing overall mental and physical health. As these findings become more widely known, people are starting to recognize that napping is not a luxury but a necessity for optimal performance.

Changing work cultures have also contributed to the shifting attitudes towards napping. With the rise of remote work and flexible schedules, individuals have more control over their daily routines. This has allowed people to incorporate napping into their daily lives and experience firsthand the positive effects it can have on their productivity. Forward-thinking companies have even started to provide nap rooms or designated spaces for employees to recharge, recognizing the value of employee well-being and the impact it has on overall productivity.

Furthermore, there is a growing understanding of the importance of self-care and prioritizing one's well-being. In a fast-paced and demanding world, people are recognizing the need to take breaks, recharge, and take care of their mental and physical health. Napping is increasingly seen as a simple yet effective way to achieve this. It is no longer considered a sign of weakness or slacking off, but rather a proactive step towards maintaining optimal performance and nurturing one's well-being.

As societal attitudes continue to shift, it is crucial to embrace the power of a nap and its potential to elevate humanity's productivity and well-being. By recognizing the benefits of napping and incorporating it into our lives, we can unlock our full potential and lead healthier, more fulfilling lives. So let us break free from the outdated notions surrounding napping and embrace the Power Nap – a transformative force that will enable us to thrive in all aspects of life.

Chapter 20. Advocating for napping rights in the workplace

In today's fast-paced and demanding world, it is no surprise that many individuals find themselves struggling to stay productive and maintain their overall well-being. From long working hours to never-ending to-do lists, it often feels like there is never enough time in the day to accomplish everything. However, what if there was a simple solution that could enhance productivity, improve mental clarity, and boost overall well-being? The answer lies in the power of napping.

We explore the transformative impact of napping on our lives and aim to advocate for napping rights in the workplace. This subchapter delves into the importance of recognizing the immense benefits of napping and how it can revolutionize the way we work.

Advocating for napping rights in the workplace

Imagine a workplace where employees are not only encouraged to take regular naps but also provided with dedicated nap spaces. Picture a culture that values rest and understands that a well-rested mind is a more focused, creative, and efficient one. By advocating for napping rights in the workplace, we can usher in a new era of productivity and well-being.

Numerous studies have shown that napping has a profound effect on cognitive function. A short power nap can improve memory, enhance problem-solving skills, and increase alertness. By incorporating napping into our work routine, we can combat the mid-afternoon slump and maintain peak performance throughout the day.

Furthermore, napping has been linked to improved mental health. Chronic sleep deprivation has been associated with increased stress, anxiety, and depression. By prioritizing napping rights in the workplace, we can create an environment that fosters mental well-being and reduces burnout.

Advocating for napping rights also promotes work-life balance. In a society that often glorifies long hours and constant hustle, it is crucial to recognize that rest is not a luxury but a necessity. By encouraging napping in the workplace, we send a message that productivity is not solely measured by the number of hours worked, but by the quality of work produced.

It's time to embrace the power of a nap and advocate for napping rights in the workplace. By redefining how we approach rest, we can unlock our full potential, enhance productivity, and improve overall well-being. Together, let us champion a new era where napping is celebrated, and the benefits of a well-rested mind are recognized as an essential component of a thriving workforce.

Incorporating Napping into Daily Life

Today, where productivity and well-being regularly take a back seat to the demands of work and personal life, finding effective ways to recharge and rejuvenate becomes essential. One powerful tool that has been overlooked for far too long is the art of napping. Welcome to the subchapter on "Incorporating Napping into Daily Life" from the groundbreaking book, "Power Nap: Elevating Humanity's Productivity and Well-being."

Napping has long been stigmatized as a sign of laziness or unproductivity. However, recent scientific studies have shown that a well-timed nap can have a profound impact on our cognitive abilities, creativity, mood, and overall performance. It's time to unlock the POWER of a NAP and harness it to enhance our lives.

So, how can you incorporate napping into your daily routine? The answer lies in understanding the science behind napping and discovering the ideal nap length and timing for your unique needs. While there is no one-size-fits-all approach, here are some tips to get you started:

1. Embrace the Power of the Power Nap: Short, 20-minute power naps have been proven to boost alertness, improve mood, and enhance

Advocating for napping rights in the workplace

cognitive function. Find a quiet and comfortable spot, set an alarm, and allow yourself to drift into a state of relaxation. You'll wake up refreshed and ready to tackle the rest of your day.

2. Schedule Naps Strategically: Pay attention to your natural energy rhythms and identify the best time for a nap. Aim for the mid-afternoon slump, typically between 2 and 4 p.m., when our energy levels naturally dip. By taking a nap during this time, you'll experience a surge of energy that will carry you through the remainder of the day.

3. Create a Nap-Friendly Environment: Designate a cozy and quiet space where you can retreat for a nap. Consider using earplugs, an eye mask, or soothing background music to create a serene atmosphere. Make it a sanctuary for rejuvenation.

4. Make Napping a Ritual: Incorporate napping into your daily routine by setting aside dedicated time for a nap. By making it a habit,

you'll reap the long-term benefits of improved focus, productivity, and overall well-being.

Remember, napping is not a luxury; it is a strategic tool to enhance your productivity and well-being. Embrace the POWER of a NAP and discover how it can transform your life. By incorporating napping into your daily routine, you will elevate your cognitive abilities, boost your mood, and unlock your true potential. Welcome to the Power Nap revolution!

Napping schedules and routines

Today, where productivity and well-being often take a back seat to constant busyness, it's crucial to recognize the power of a nap. Napping has been scientifically proven to have numerous benefits for our physical, mental, and emotional well-being. By incorporating a well-thought-out napping schedule and routine into our lives, we can unlock the potential of the Power Nap and elevate our overall productivity and well-being.

A napping schedule refers to the predetermined times during the day when we allocate a specific period for napping. It's essential to establish a routine that aligns with our natural circadian rhythm. Our bodies have an innate tendency to feel drowsy in the mid-afternoon, making it an ideal time for a power nap. By scheduling a short nap during this period, we can combat the notorious afternoon slump and recharge our energy levels.

Consistency is key when it comes to napping schedules. By adhering to a routine, we train our bodies to anticipate and prepare for the restorative benefits of a nap. The duration of a nap is equally important. Short power naps, ranging from 10 to 30 minutes, can provide an instant boost in alertness and mental clarity without leaving us feeling groggy or interfering with nighttime sleep. However, for those who have more time available or need extra restoration, longer naps of 60 to 90 minutes (about 1 and a half hours) can help enhance creativity, memory consolidation, and overall cognitive function.

Advocating for napping rights in the workplace

To make the most out of a nap, creating a conducive environment is vital. Find a quiet and comfortable space where you can relax without distraction. Dimming the lights or using an eye mask can help signal to your body that it's time to rest. Consider using soothing sounds or calming music to enhance relaxation and facilitate a quicker transition into sleep. Additionally, incorporating relaxation techniques such as deep breathing or meditation can help clear the mind and induce a more restful nap.

By embracing the power of a nap and establishing a well-planned napping schedule and routine, we can tap into the incredible benefits that napping offers. From improved productivity and enhanced cognitive function to reduced stress levels and increased well-being, napping truly has the potential to elevate humanity's overall quality of life. So, let's prioritize self-care, embrace the Power Nap, and unlock our full potential through the simple act of napping.

Chapter 21. Napping habits for different age groups

In "Power Nap: Elevating Humanity's Productivity and Well-being," we explore the fascinating and often overlooked world of napping habits for different age groups. As we delve into the power of a nap, it becomes evident that understanding how different age groups can benefit from this practice is essential for unlocking our full potential as individuals and as a society.

Infants and toddlers are known for their frequent napping habits. These little ones require a significant amount of sleep, and daytime naps are crucial for their growth and development. Parents and caregivers play a vital role in establishing healthy nap routines, ensuring that these young minds get the rest they need to thrive.

Napping habits for different age groups

Moving on to children and adolescents, napping habits may change as they grow older. While some children may outgrow their need for daytime naps, others may continue to benefit from short power naps to recharge their energy levels. As they juggle school, extracurricular activities, and social interactions, naps can help them stay focused, improve memory retention, and enhance overall cognitive function.

Adults, on the other hand, often find it challenging to prioritize napping in their busy lives. However, research suggests that incorporating short naps into our daily routine can yield significant benefits. Napping can help combat afternoon drowsiness, improve mood and overall well-being, and enhance cognitive performance. Whether it's a quick power nap during a lunch break or a longer restorative nap on the weekends, adults can tap into the rejuvenating power of napping to optimize their productivity and well-being.

The elderly population also stands to gain from napping habits tailored to their specific needs.

Napping habits for different age groups

As we age, our sleep patterns may change, leading to fragmented nighttime sleep. Incorporating regular naps can help compensate for this and improve sleep quality. Napping can also reduce the risk of age-related cognitive decline, boost memory, and enhance overall mental sharpness.

Understanding the napping habits of different age groups allows us to harness the power of a nap to elevate humanity's productivity and well-being. By recognizing the unique benefits that napping offers individuals at each stage of life, we can foster healthier sleep habits, improve cognitive function, and ultimately enhance our quality of life.

So, whether you're a parent guiding your child's nap routine, an adult seeking an energy boost, or an elderly individual looking to improve sleep quality, remember that a well-timed nap can be the key to unlocking your fullest potential. Embrace the power of a nap, and watch as it transforms your life, one restful moment at a time.

Napping habits for different age groups

Napping as a family activity

In our fast-paced and busy lives, finding quality time to spend with our loved ones can be challenging. However, there is one activity that can help us reconnect, relax, and rejuvenate together – napping as a family. While napping is often seen as an individual activity, it has the power to bring families closer and enhance their overall well-being.

The POWER of a NAP extends beyond the physical benefits. When families nap together, they create a safe and nurturing environment where everyone can unwind and recharge. It allows members to escape from the stresses of daily life and enter a realm of tranquility as a unit. As individuals, we frequently struggle to find the time to take care of ourselves, but when we nap together, we prioritize our collective health and happiness.

Napping as a family activity fosters stronger bonds among loved ones. It encourages communication, trust, and a sense of togetherness. By synchronizing our sleep schedules, we align our bodies and minds, creating a harmonious atmosphere where everyone can let go of their worries and simply be present with each other. It is during these moments of vulnerability and relaxation that we deepen our connections, building a foundation of love, support, and understanding.

Furthermore, napping together promotes better sleep hygiene. As we share our sleep routines, we can help each other establish healthier habits, ensuring that everyone gets the rest they need. By setting aside time for family naps, we prioritize our mental and physical well-being, leading to increased productivity, improved mood, and reduced stress levels.

Napping as a family activity also encourages mindfulness and self-care. In a world that glorifies busyness, taking the time to slow down and rest together can be a revolutionary act. It sends a powerful message to our children, teaching them the importance of self-care and balance. By embracing napping as a family, we demonstrate that rest is not a sign of weakness, but a crucial element in leading a fulfilling and productive life.

Summary, napping as a family activity has the potential to transform our lives. By prioritizing our collective well-being, fostering stronger bonds, and promoting healthier sleep habits, we elevate our productivity and overall happiness. Let us embrace the POWER of a NAP and make it a cherished activity that brings us closer together as families, reminding us of the importance of rest, relaxation, and connection in our lives.

Napping Etiquette and Best Practices

Introduction:In our fast-paced and demanding world, it is no surprise that many individuals find themselves struggling to maintain optimal productivity and well-being. Fortunately, there is a powerful tool available to all of humanity: the art of napping. Napping has been scientifically proven to enhance productivity, creativity, and overall well-being. However, to fully harness the POWER of a NAP, it is crucial to understand the importance of napping etiquette and best practices.

Respect Personal Boundaries: When it comes to napping, it is essential to respect personal boundaries. If you are in a shared space, ensure that you are considerate of others who may also need a nap. Avoid unnecessary noise or disruptions and be mindful of the time you spend napping to allow others the opportunity to rejuvenate as well.

Create a Restful Environment:

To optimize the benefits of a nap, it is crucial to create a restful environment. Find a quiet and comfortable space where you can relax and unwind. Dim the lights or use a sleep mask to block out any excess light. Consider using earplugs or playing soothing music to drown out disturbing noises. By creating an atmosphere conducive to relaxation, you will enhance the quality of your nap and maximize its effect.

Set an Alarm: One common concern with napping is the fear of oversleeping and disrupting the daily routine. To avoid this, it is essential to set an alarm before you drift off. By doing so, you can ensure that your nap remains within a reasonable timeframe, typically ranging between 20 and 30 minutes. This duration allows you to reap the benefits of restorative sleep without entering a deep sleep cycle, which can lead to grogginess upon awakening.

Practice Consistency: Consistency is key when it comes to napping. Establish a regular schedule for napping, preferably during the mid-afternoon, when the body naturally experiences a dip in energy levels. By consistently incorporating naps into your routine, you will train your body to anticipate and benefit from this designated rest period, leading to improved overall productivity and well-being.

Napping etiquette and best practices are essential to fully harness the POWER of a NAP. By respecting personal boundaries, creating a restful environment, setting an alarm, and practicing consistency, you can optimize the benefits of napping. Embracing this powerful tool will elevate your productivity and well-being, allowing you to navigate life's challenges with renewed energy and focus. So go ahead, take that nap and unlock the potential within you!

Proper nap duration and timing guidelines

Napping has long been viewed as a luxury or a sign of laziness. However, recent scientific research has revealed the incredible benefits of a well-timed and properly executed nap. In this subchapter, we will explore the guidelines for the ideal nap duration and timing, empowering humanity to harness the POWER of a nap for enhanced productivity and well-being.

The duration of a nap plays a crucial role in determining its effectiveness. Short power naps, lasting between 10 and 20 minutes, are ideal for boosting alertness and improving cognitive function. These quick naps can help combat the post-lunch dip, providing a burst of energy to tackle the rest of the day. By keeping the nap short, you avoid entering deeper stages of sleep, preventing grogginess upon waking.

For those seeking a more profound rejuvenation, a longer nap of 60 to 90 minutes (about 1 and a half hours) is recommended. This duration allows for a complete sleep cycle, including both light and deep sleep. This type of nap is especially beneficial for memory consolidation, creativity enhancement, and emotional restoration. However, it's important to note that longer naps may lead to sleep inertia upon awakening, which can be mitigated by allowing a few minutes for transition before engaging in demanding tasks.

Napping habits for different age groups

Timing is just as essential as duration when it comes to maximizing the benefits of a nap. The optimal time for a power nap is between 1 pm to 3 pm, aligning with the natural circadian rhythm of the human body. This period is commonly associated with the post-lunch slump, where productivity tends to decline. A well-timed nap during this window can counteract the dip, leaving individuals feeling revitalized and ready to tackle the remainder of the day.

However, it's essential to adapt the timing to personal preferences and lifestyle. Some individuals may find it more beneficial to nap earlier or later in the day, depending on their sleep patterns and daily routines. Experimentation and self-awareness are key to finding the ideal timing that complements individual needs.

Summary, understanding the proper guidelines for nap duration and timing is crucial for unlocking the full potential of the POWER of a nap. Whether it's a short power nap to combat fatigue or a longer nap for enhanced creativity and emotional well-being, mastering the art of napping can elevate productivity and overall well-being for humanity. So, embrace the nap revolution and experience the transformative effects it can have on your life.

Chapter 22. Napping etiquette in public spaces

In our fast-paced world, finding time to rest and recharge has become increasingly important. One powerful tool that has gained recognition for its ability to enhance productivity and well-being is the art of napping. The POWER of a NAP is undeniable, but what about napping etiquette in public spaces? How can we ensure that our napping practices are considerate and respectful to others?

First, it is crucial to be mindful of the surrounding space. Public spaces are shared by many, and it is essential to be respectful of others' needs and boundaries. When choosing a spot to take a nap, opt for areas designated for relaxation or where napping is accepted. Avoid areas that may disrupt others, such as busy walkways or dining areas.

Napping etiquette in public spaces

Noise is another significant factor to consider. While some people may prefer a quiet environment to nap, others may find comfort in white noise or ambient sounds. Be aware of the volume of any devices you may use, such as headphones or white noise machines, to ensure they do not disturb those around you. If you are in a public space with designated quiet zones, respect the silence and refrain from engaging in loud conversations or phone calls.

Furthermore, be mindful of your personal hygiene and the odors you may carry. It is essential to maintain cleanliness and avoid strong scents that may be overwhelming to others. Perfumes, colognes, or even the smell of food can be disruptive to those nearby. Consider using unscented products or minimizing the use of strong fragrances to create a pleasant environment for everyone.

Respecting personal boundaries is paramount. Avoid invading others' personal space by keeping your belongings contained and ensuring that you are not encroaching on someone else's designated area. If someone is already napping nearby, give them ample space and avoid any unnecessary disturbances.

Lastly, be conscious of the duration of your nap. While a quick power nap can be rejuvenating, extended napping periods may not be suitable for public spaces. If you feel the need for a more extended nap, consider finding a designated rest area or returning to the comfort of your space.

By adhering to these napping etiquette guidelines, we can foster a harmonious environment in public spaces. The POWER of a NAP should not come at the expense of others' comfort. Let us cultivate a culture of respect and consideration, allowing everyone to reap the benefits of rest and rejuvenation while maintaining the well-being of humanity.

Creating nap-friendly environments in schools and workplaces

Today, where productivity is highly valued, and stress levels are soaring, finding ways to enhance our well-being and performance has become paramount. One often overlooked solution that has a profound impact on our productivity and overall health is the power of a nap. Napping has been proven to boost creativity, increase focus, and improve memory retention. Understanding the immense benefits of napping, it becomes crucial to create nap-friendly environments in schools and workplaces.

In schools, where students are expected to absorb vast amounts of information, napping can be a game-changer. By incorporating designated nap areas, schools can provide students with a space to recharge and consolidate their learning. These nap areas can be designed to be peaceful, quiet, and equipped with comfortable furniture. Dimmed lighting and soft music can further enhance the relaxation experience. Educators can encourage students to utilize these nap areas during designated break times, helping them to rejuvenate and return to their studies with renewed energy and focus.

Similarly, workplaces can greatly benefit from nap-friendly environments. Many employees experience midday fatigue, leading to decreased productivity and creativity. By providing designated areas for napping, companies can unlock the potential of their workforce. Nap rooms or pods can be created, allowing employees to take short power naps during their lunch breaks or whenever they feel their energy levels dip. These spaces should be designed to be calm, quiet, and equipped with comfortable seating. Employers should also encourage nap breaks, as they have been shown to enhance alertness and problem-solving skills, leading to increased efficiency and job satisfaction.

Creating nap-friendly environments in schools and workplaces is not just about providing physical spaces; it also involves cultivating a culture that values rest and recognizes the importance of mental well-being. Leaders and educators should educate others about the benefits of napping and encourage its incorporation into daily routines. By fostering an environment that prioritizes rest and rejuvenation, schools and workplaces can enhance productivity, creativity, and overall well-being.

Summary, integrating nap-friendly environments in schools and workplaces can have a profound impact on individuals' productivity, creativity, and overall well-being. By providing designated spaces for napping and fostering a culture that values rest, we can unlock the true potential of humanity. Let us embrace the power of a nap and create environments that elevate productivity and well-being for all.

Chapter 23. The Future of Napping

In this subchapter, we delve into the fascinating world of napping technology and innovation, exploring how advancements in this field are transforming the way we rest and rejuvenate. As we unlock the power of a nap, we are witnessing a revolution in productivity and well-being that has the potential to elevate humanity to new heights.

The POWER of a NAP has been recognized for centuries, but it is only in recent years that technology has caught up with this ancient practice. Today, we have access to a plethora of innovative tools and gadgets designed to enhance our napping experience.

One remarkable innovation is the development of smart mattresses and sleep tracking devices. Equipped with sensors and advanced algorithms, these mattresses can monitor our sleep patterns, detect when we are in a light sleep stage, and wake us up at the optimal time, ensuring we feel refreshed and energized after a nap.

Additionally, wearable devices such as smartwatches have gained popularity in the field of napping technology. These devices track our sleep and offer guided meditation and relaxation exercises to help us unwind and fall asleep faster. With features like gentle vibrating alarms, they ensure we wake up smoothly, without disrupting our sleep cycle.

Another exciting advancement is the introduction of nap pods and sleep pods in various workplaces, airports, and public spaces. These cozy, futuristic capsules provide a quiet and comfortable environment for quick power naps, allowing individuals to recharge and boost their cognitive abilities. Some pods even incorporate ambient lighting, soothing sounds, and aromatherapy to create the perfect nap-inducing atmosphere.

Furthermore, virtual reality (VR) technology has made its way into the napping realm. VR headsets offer immersive experiences, transporting users to serene landscapes or tranquil environments, promoting relaxation and facilitating deep sleep. This innovation has the potential to revolutionize the way we nap, providing a personalized and customizable escape from the stresses of daily life.

As humanity embraces napping technology and innovation, we are witnessing a transformation in our productivity and well-being. The integration of smart devices, sleep tracking tools, nap pods, and VR technology has opened a new world of possibilities for achieving optimal rest and rejuvenation. By harnessing the POWER of a NAP through these advancements, we can unlock our full potential and elevate our overall quality of life.

Advancements in sleep tracking devices

Today, the importance of quality sleep cannot be overstated. As humanity strives for higher

The Future of Napping

productivity and overall well-being, it has become crucial to monitor and optimize our sleep patterns. Thankfully, advancements in sleep tracking devices have revolutionized the way we understand and improve our sleep.

Sleep tracking devices are wearable gadgets that utilize innovative technology to monitor various aspects of our sleep, providing valuable insights into our sleep quality and duration. These devices have come a long way in recent years, evolving from simple wristbands that tracked basic metrics to sophisticated smartwatches and futuristic headbands capable of analyzing brainwaves.

One of the key advancements in sleep tracking devices is their ability to measure sleep stages. Traditionally, sleep was divided into two stages: rapid eye movement (REM) and non-rapid eye movement (NREM). However, with the advent of advanced sensors and algorithms, modern sleep trackers can now accurately detect and differentiate between light sleep, deep sleep, REM sleep, and even micro-arousals. This level of detail allows individuals to understand their sleep architecture better and make necessary adjustments to improve sleep quality.

Another significant improvement is the integration of artificial intelligence (AI) capabilities into sleep tracking devices. AI algorithms can analyze vast amounts of sleep data, detect patterns, and provide personalized recommendations to enhance sleep. These recommendations can range from adjusting bedtime routines, optimizing sleep schedules, or even suggesting specific sleep aids based on an individual's unique sleep patterns and habits.

Furthermore, sleep tracking devices have become increasingly user-friendly and accessible to a wider audience. They now offer intuitive interfaces, seamless integration with smartphones, and comprehensive data visualization. This empowers individuals to take control of their sleep health and make informed decisions to optimize their overall well-being.

The POWER of a NAP, a book dedicated to elevating humanity's productivity and well-being, recognizes the significance of sleep tracking devices in achieving these goals. By leveraging the advancements in sleep tracking technology, individuals can unlock the power of a nap, ensuring they reap the maximum benefits of restorative sleep.

In summary, advancements in sleep tracking devices have transformed the way we understand and improve our sleep. With their ability to measure sleep stages, integration of AI capabilities, and user-friendly interfaces, these devices have become invaluable tools for enhancing sleep quality and overall well-being. By embracing the power of a nap and utilizing these innovative devices, humanity can embark on a journey towards elevated productivity and optimal health.

Napping aids and accessories

Napping aids and accessories have become increasingly popular in recent years, as

The Future of Napping

increasing numbers of people recognize the power and benefits of a well-timed nap. In this subchapter, we will explore the various tools and items that can enhance your napping experience, allowing you to reap the full potential of a rejuvenating nap.

One of the most essential napping aids is a comfortable pillow. Investing in a high-quality pillow that supports your neck and head can make all the difference in achieving a restful nap. There are several types of pillows available, such as memory foam, shredded memory foam, and down pillows, each offering unique levels of comfort and support. Finding the right pillow for you is crucial in creating a cozy and inviting nap environment.

Another popular napping accessory is a sleep mask. Sleep masks block out light and help create a dark and peaceful environment, promoting deeper sleep. They are especially useful for those who struggle with falling asleep during the day or in bright environments. Sleep masks are typically made from soft materials and are adjustable to fit different head sizes, ensuring a snug and comfortable fit.

For individuals who prefer a more sensory-focused nap experience, there are napping aids that incorporate soothing sounds and scents. White noise machines or smartphone apps can produce calming sounds like ocean waves or rainfall, creating a peaceful ambiance conducive to napping. Additionally, essential oils or aromatherapy diffusers can be used to infuse the air with relaxing scents like lavender or chamomile, further enhancing the tranquility of your nap.

Lastly, consider incorporating a weighted blanket into your napping routine. These blankets provide gentle pressure and mimic the feeling of being hugged, inducing a sense of relaxation and security. The deep touch pressure stimulation from a weighted blanket has been shown to reduce anxiety and promote better sleep, making it an ideal addition to your napping arsenal.

The Future of Napping

Remember, napping is a powerful tool for increasing productivity and overall well-being. By carefully selecting the right aids and accessories, you can optimize your napping experience and harness the full potential of a restorative nap. Whether it's a comfortable pillow, a sleep mask, soothing sounds, or a weighted blanket, these tools can transform your nap into a rejuvenating and transformative practice. So, embrace the power of a nap and give yourself the gift of enhanced productivity and well-being.

Emerging trends in nap-related technologies

In the fast-paced world we live in, finding time to rest and rejuvenate has become increasingly challenging. However, emerging trends in nap-related technologies are revolutionizing the way we approach relaxation, leading to a profound impact on productivity and well-being. These innovations are a result of extensive research and the understanding of the POWER of a NAP.

The Future of Napping

One of the most exciting advancements in nap-related technologies is the development of smart sleepwear. These intelligent garments are embedded with sensors that monitor your sleep patterns, body temperature, and heart rate. By analyzing this data, they can create personalized sleep profiles and provide feedback to optimize your napping experience. Imagine slipping into comfortable sleepwear that enhances your nap and ensures you wake up feeling refreshed and energized.

Another trend that is transforming nap-related technologies is the rise of brainwave stimulation devices. These cutting-edge devices use gentle electrical impulses or sound waves to stimulate specific brain regions, inducing a state of deep relaxation and promoting restful sleep. With the help of these devices, nap enthusiasts can now achieve a more profound level of rest in a shorter amount of time, maximizing the benefits of their power nap.

Virtual reality (VR) is also making its way into the world of napping. VR headsets, combined with soothing audio and visual simulations, create immersive environments that transport individuals to tranquil and peaceful settings. Whether it's a serene beach or a tranquil forest, these virtual experiences help individuals relax and reduce stress and anxiety levels, allowing for a more restorative nap experience.

The integration of artificial intelligence (AI) in nap-related technologies is yet another emerging trend. AI-powered nap assistants can analyze a range of factors like sleep patterns, stress levels, and daily routines to generate personalized nap schedules. These assistants can also offer valuable insights and tips to optimize nap duration and timing, further enhancing the benefits of a nap and improving overall well-being.

As nap-related technologies continue to evolve, the possibilities for enhancing productivity and well-being are limitless. The POWER of a NAP is being harnessed through smart sleepwear, brainwave stimulation devices, virtual reality, and AI-powered nap assistants. These advancements are empowering humanity to reclaim their energy, boost cognitive performance, and improve the overall quality of life.

It is essential for individuals and society to embrace these emerging trends in nap-related technologies. By recognizing the importance of rest and implementing these innovations, we can elevate our productivity, well-being, and ultimately achieve a more balanced and fulfilling life.

Napping in a Hyper-Connected World

In today's hyper-connected world, where we are constantly bombarded with notifications, emails, and social media updates, it has become increasingly challenging to find moments of peace and relaxation. The constant demands on our attention and the pressure to be constantly productive to have taken a toll on our mental and physical well-being.

Enter the POWER of a NAP – a simple yet transformative practice that can elevate

The Future of Napping

humanity's productivity and well-being. Napping, often overlooked and undervalued, holds the key to unlocking our full potential in this fast-paced, hyper-connected world.

In a society that glorifies busyness, the idea of taking a nap may seem counterintuitive. But the truth is, regular napping has been scientifically proven to enhance our cognitive abilities, memory retention, creativity, and overall performance. It is not only a luxury, but a necessity for our minds and bodies to function optimally.

When we nap, our brain enters a state of restorative sleep, allowing it to consolidate memories, process information, and rejuvenate. This period of rest can be a notable change, as it enhances our ability to focus, make sound decisions, and be more efficient in our tasks. The POWER of a NAP lies in its ability to recharge our mental batteries, enabling us to tackle challenges with renewed vigor and clarity.

Moreover, napping offers a respite from the constant noise and distractions of our hyper-connected world. It provides an opportunity to disconnect, unwind, and reconnect with us. By intentionally carving out time for a nap, we are prioritizing our well-being and reclaiming control over our lives.

Imagine a world where napping becomes a cultural norm, where workplaces and educational institutions recognize the value of rest and provide dedicated spaces for napping. The Power Nap can revolutionize our society, not only by enhancing productivity, but also by fostering a healthier and more balanced lifestyle.

It is time for humanity to embrace the POWER of a NAP and unlock its incredible potential. By incorporating regular napping into our daily routines, we can reclaim our focus, creativity, and overall well-being. Let us break free from the shackles of constant connectivity, and instead, embrace the transformative power of a nap. It is time to elevate humanity's productivity and well-being – one nap at a time.

The Future of Napping

Napping strategies for digital detoxification

In today's fast-paced and technology-driven world, it has become increasingly difficult for humanity to disconnect from the digital realm and find moments of genuine relaxation. The constant bombardment of emails, social media notifications, and work-related demands can take a toll on our productivity and overall well-being. However, there is a simple yet powerful solution that can help us detoxify from our digital dependencies – napping.

The POWER of a NAP is a concept that emphasizes the transformative effects of a well-timed and intentional nap. It is not just about catching a few minutes of shut eye; it is about using napping as a strategic tool to rejuvenate our minds, improve our cognitive abilities, and ultimately enhance our productivity and well-being.

To effectively use napping as a strategy for digital detoxification, it is essential to follow a few key strategies. Firstly, setting boundaries is crucial. Designate specific periods of the day when you will disconnect from all digital devices, allowing yourself the opportunity to rest and recharge. This could be during lunch breaks or in the late afternoon when energy levels tend to dip.

Creating a conducive environment for napping is equally important. Find a quiet and comfortable space, away from the distractions of technology. Dim the lights, play soothing music, or use white noise machines to drown out any external disturbances. These small adjustments can greatly enhance the quality of your nap and facilitate deeper relaxation.

Timing your nap appropriately is another critical aspect. The optimal duration for a power nap is typically between 10 and 30 minutes. A shorter nap can provide a quick energy boost, while a longer nap may leave you feeling groggy and disrupt your sleep cycle.

In addition to these strategies, it is essential to prioritize consistency and make napping a regular part of your routine. By incorporating naps into your daily schedule, you will gradually train your body to recognize and respond to these moments of relaxation, making it easier to disconnect from the digital world.

Remember, napping is not a sign of laziness or unproductivity; it is a proactive step towards self-care and digital detoxification. Embracing the POWER of a NAP can have a profound impact on your overall well-being, helping you cultivate a healthier relationship with technology and enhancing your productivity in the process.

So, take a break, find a cozy spot, and allow yourself the luxury of a rejuvenating nap. Your mind, body, and productivity levels will thank you for it.

Napping's role in managing technology-induced stress

In today's fast-paced, technology-driven world, stress has become an unwelcome companion for many individuals. The constant barrage of

The Future of Napping

emails, social media notifications, and endless streams of information can leave us feeling overwhelmed and mentally exhausted. Fortunately, there is a simple and effective solution to combat this modern-day stress: napping.

Napping has long been associated with relaxation and rejuvenation, but its role in managing technology-induced stress is often overlooked. When we are constantly plugged into our devices, our minds are bombarded with information, multitasking becomes the norm, and our brains are on high alert. The result? Burnout, decreased productivity, and a decline in overall well-being.

Taking a nap during the day can serve as a reset button for our brains. It allows us to disconnect from the digital world and gives our minds the much-needed break they deserve. Just a short power nap can help alleviate stress, improve cognitive function, and boost creativity.

One of the key benefits of napping is its ability to reduce cortisol levels, the hormone responsible for stress. When we are constantly exposed to the demands of technology, our cortisol levels can skyrocket, leading to feelings of anxiety and tension. By taking a nap, we give our bodies a chance to recalibrate and bring these levels back down to a healthier range, promoting a sense of calm and relaxation.

Furthermore, napping can enhance our cognitive abilities. Studies have shown that a brief nap can improve memory, attention span, and problem-solving skills. By allowing our brains to rest and recharge, we are better equipped to handle the challenges that technology presents us with.

Additionally, napping can unlock our creativity. When we are constantly bombarded with information and distractions, it can be difficult to encourage creative thinking and come up with innovative solutions. A nap provides us with an opportunity to enter a state of relaxed wakefulness, where ideas can flow freely, and our creative juices can flourish.

In a world that glorifies hustle and constant connectivity, embracing the power of a nap may seem counterintuitive. However, prioritizing rest and well-being is crucial for maintaining productivity and overall happiness. So, the next time you feel overwhelmed by technology-induced stress, consider taking a nap. You'll be amazed at the transformative effect it can have on your mind, body, and soul. Embrace the Power Nap and elevate your productivity and well-being to new heights.

Balancing productivity and rest in the modern age

Today, where technology has permeated every aspect of our lives, finding a balance between productivity and rest has become an elusive challenge. As we strive to achieve more, we often overlook the fundamental need for rest, leading to burnout and a decline in overall well-being. In this subchapter, we will explore the crucial importance of striking a balance between productivity and rest, and how The Power Nap can revolutionize our approach to both.

The modern age has witnessed a relentless pursuit of productivity, with individuals striving to maximize their output in every aspect of their lives. While this ambition is commendable, it frequently comes at the expense of rest and rejuvenation. However, research has proven repeatedly that productivity and rest are not mutually exclusive but rather interdependent. The POWER of a NAP lies in its ability to enhance both productivity and well-being simultaneously.

In our quest for optimal productivity, we regularly neglect the fact that our brains and bodies require regular periods of rest to perform at their best. Scientific studies have shown that short periods of rest, such as a power nap, can significantly improve cognitive function, memory retention, and creativity. The Power Nap taps into this potential, allowing individuals to recharge and refocus, leading to heightened productivity levels.

Moreover, the subchapter delves into the detrimental effects of chronic sleep deprivation, a prevalent issue in the modern age. Lack of sleep not only impairs cognitive abilities but also negatively impacts physical health, emotional well-being, and overall productivity. By incorporating strategic rest periods, such as power naps, into our daily routines, we can mitigate the harmful consequences of sleep deprivation and achieve a harmonious balance between productivity and rest.

Power Nap further explores the concept of intentional rest, emphasizing the importance of quality over quantity. It advocates for mindful rest breaks that allow individuals to detach from the constant demands of technology and engage in activities that promote relaxation and rejuvenation. By incorporating such intentional rest periods, individuals can rewire their brains for enhanced focus, creativity, and overall well-being.

Summary, the subchapter "Balancing Productivity and Rest in the Modern Age" sheds light on the urgent need to strike a harmonious equilibrium between productivity and rest. Through The Power Nap, individuals can harness the power of intentional rest breaks and power naps to enhance their productivity, cognitive function, and overall well-being. By embracing the POWER of a NAP, humanity can elevate its productivity levels while simultaneously prioritizing rest, ultimately leading to a healthier, happier, and more productive future.

The Future of Napping

Napping as a Catalyst for Societal Change

In this fast-paced world, where productivity and well-being are often neglected, there is a powerful yet underrated tool that has the potential to revolutionize our lives – napping. Yes, you read that right! Napping has the power to become a catalyst for societal change, transforming the way we work, think, and live. Welcome to the world of "Power Nap: Elevating Humanity's Productivity and Well-being."

For centuries, napping has been an integral part of our natural sleep-wake cycle. However, in modern society, it has been largely stigmatized as a sign of laziness or unproductivity. But what if we told you that napping could be the key to unlocking our true potential?

"The POWER of a NAP" lies in its ability to rejuvenate our minds and bodies, allowing us to recharge and refocus. Studies have shown that a short power nap can increase alertness, improve memory and cognitive function, and enhance creativity. Imagine a society where individuals

The Future of Napping

are not constantly burnt out, but instead are energized and motivated to tackle challenges head-on.

By embracing the power of napping, we can transform our workplaces into more productive and efficient environments. Rather than pushing ourselves to the brink of exhaustion, we can create a culture that values rest and recognizes the importance of mental and physical well-being. Companies that encourage napping as a regular practice have reported higher employee satisfaction, decreased absenteeism, and increased overall productivity. It's time to redefine success and acknowledge that true productivity is not measured by the number of hours spent working, but by the quality and impact of our output.

But the Power Nap doesn't stop at the workplace. It has the potential to revolutionize our education system, healthcare, and even our relationships. Imagine schools where students are given designated nap times to consolidate their learning and improve their focus. Picture hospitals where doctors and nurses can take short naps to prevent medical errors caused by fatigue. Envision a society where couples and families prioritize rest and rejuvenation, fostering stronger bonds and healthier relationships.

Humanity, it's time to awaken to the transformative power of napping. Let's break free from the chains of societal norms and embrace a new way of living – one where napping is not only accepted but celebrated. Together, we can create a world where productivity and well-being go hand in hand, where napping becomes the catalyst for societal change. Are you ready to experience "The Power Nap?"

The Potential Impact of Widespread Napping on Productivity

Introduction:In this chapter, we will explore the potential impact of widespread napping on productivity. While napping has long been associated with laziness or unproductivity, recent scientific research has challenged this notion, highlighting the transformative power of a nap on overall well-being and productivity. By understanding the true potential of naps, we can unlock a new level of productivity and well-being for humanity.

The Science Behind Napping: Numerous studies have revealed the positive effects of napping on cognitive function, memory consolidation, and creativity. Napping has been shown to improve alertness, enhance problem-solving abilities, and boost mood. As a result, individuals who incorporate naps into their daily routines are better equipped to handle challenges and make sound decisions, ultimately leading to increased productivity.

The Power Nap how it makes us feel

Beyond mental benefits, napping also impacts physical health. Regular napping has been linked to reduced cardiovascular risks, lower blood pressure, and decreased stress levels. By promoting relaxation and reducing fatigue, napping contributes to a healthier lifestyle, enabling individuals to approach their work and personal lives with greater energy and vigor.

Napping and Innovation: Napping enhances productivity on an individual level and has the potential to foster innovation and creativity across various industries. Companies that embrace napping as part of their culture have reported increased employee creativity, problem-solving abilities, and overall job satisfaction. By providing designated nap spaces or implementing nap policies, organizations can harness the power of napping to drive innovation and achieve remarkable breakthroughs.

Overcoming the Stigma: Despite the growing body of evidence supporting the benefits of napping, there still exists a stigma surrounding its practice. Many individuals feel guilty or fear judgment for taking a nap during the day. However, it is crucial to recognize that napping is not a sign of weakness or laziness, but rather a strategic tool for enhancing productivity and well-being. By overcoming this stigma, society can embrace napping as a legitimate and powerful approach to boosting productivity.

Conclusion: The potential impact of widespread napping on productivity is immense. Incorporating naps into our daily routines can lead to improved cognitive function, enhanced physical health, and increased creativity. By recognizing the transformative power of napping, we can unlock humanity's full potential, elevating productivity and well-being for all. It is time for us to embrace "The Power Nap" and harness the power of a nap to revolutionize our lives and the world we live in. Together, let us redefine productivity and create a more balanced and fulfilling future.

Napping as a Mechanism for Work-Life Balance

Many people struggle to find a healthy balance between their work and personal lives. Long work hours, job stress, and lack of sleep can take a toll on mental and physical health. However, research shows that taking short naps during the workday may help improve productivity, cognitive functioning, and overall well-being. Implementing napping as part of the workplace culture could be an effective strategy for achieving better work-life balance.

Benefits of Napping

Several studies have uncovered a wide range of benefits associated with brief daytime naps. A NASA study found that a 26-minute nap improved pilots' performance by 34% and alertness by 54%

(1). Another study showed that naps as short as 10 minutes enhanced cognitive performance and mood (2). Participants who took a nap were less impulsive and had improved memory recall compared to non-nappers.

Napping may also boost learning. A study by the University of California, San Diego examined how naps affect the brain's ability to retain visual information. Participants took a 60–90-minute nap after watching an educational video. Researchers found that the nappers retained the information better than participants who stayed awake, likely due to memory consolidation that occurred during sleep (3). In addition to cognitive benefits, napping offers numerous health advantages. Research shows that people who take afternoon naps have lower blood pressure than non-nappers, reducing the risk for heart disease (4). Napping may also help fend off depression and anxiety. One study found that university students who napped at least twice a week had fewer symptoms of depression than those who napped less often (5). The refreshing sleep charges the brain's batteries and fights mental fatigue.

Impact on Work Performance

The cognitive and emotional benefits of naps translate into improved work performance. Well-timed naps have been shown to boost productivity and problem-solving skills. In one study, participants completed a visual task before and after a 60-minute afternoon nap. The nappers demonstrated a 20% improvement in performance after waking up (6). Their non-napping counterparts showed no such jump in productivity.

Research also indicates that naps help maintain focus and alertness throughout the workday. Fatigue sets in naturally during the late afternoon, typically between 2-4 pm. This lag in energy hinders our ability to concentrate. However, a short 20–30-minute nap prevents the post-lunch dip in performance (7). Employees avoid the brain fog that typically follows lunch and remain effective for the rest of their shift.

Furthermore, brief naps help employees persevere through challenging cognitive tasks. A study by researchers at the University of Michigan found that subjects who napped for an hour were able to tolerate frustration better when trying to solve an impossible puzzle. They spent nearly 50% more time working on the puzzle than non-nappers (8).

Implementing Napping Policies

The Future of Napping

To reap the benefits of napping, companies should consider allowing and encouraging brief daytime naps. Napping spaces outfitted with reclining chairs, eye masks, and earplugs can promote sleep. Providing employees with 30-minute power naps may optimize productivity.

Management could also implement flexible "nap time" policies. Allowing employees to take short 20-minute naps when needed is a cost-effective way to boost energy levels. Nap opportunities may be especially beneficial for jobs requiring sustained concentration and alertness, like air traffic controllers, truck drivers, and pilots.

Some companies, like Google, have already created nap-friendly work environments. Google offers futuristic napping pods where employees can get some shut eye and return to work refreshed. Research shows that workplaces that provide nap opportunities have higher productivity and job satisfaction (9).

The Future of Napping

However, napping may not work for every corporate culture. Companies should survey employees to gauge interest and identify optimal nap times that align with workflow. Effective implementation requires buy-in from management and a clear nap policy.

Research strongly supports the notion that brief midday naps offer cognitive and health benefits that translate into improved job performance. Allowing flexible nap times may boost productivity, focus, and learning. Companies looking to achieve a better work-life balance for employees should consider incorporating napping opportunities during the workday. Brief naps leave workers feeling rejuvenated and ready to perform at full capacity, while also supporting personal health and wellness.

Chapter 24: Embracing the Nap Revolution: A Brighter Future for Well-being

In our fast-paced, always-on world, the concept of a good night's sleep has become an elusive dream for many. We find ourselves caught in a relentless cycle of work, stress, and exhaustion, with little time to recharge our batteries. But what if the solution to our modern malaise has been right under our noses all along? Enter the nap: a powerful tool that has the potential to transform not just our personal lives, but society.

For too long, napping has been unfairly maligned, dismissed as a sign of laziness or a lack of ambition. But the truth is far more compelling. Innovative research has revealed that napping is not a luxury, but a necessity – a vital key to unlocking our full potential. A short

Napping's role in redefining societal norms around sleep

20-minute nap can work wonders, sharpening our focus, boosting our creativity, and enhancing our memory. It's like a supercharged coffee break for the brain, without the jitters or the crash.

But the benefits of napping extend far beyond the realm of productivity. When we nap, we give our bodies and minds a chance to rest, recharge, and heal. We reduce stress, lower our blood pressure, and fortify our immune systems. In a world where burnout and chronic stress have become all too common, napping offers a lifeline – a simple yet profound way to prioritize our well-being and reclaim our zest for life.

Imagine a future where napping is not just accepted but celebrated – where companies provide cozy nap rooms as a standard employee benefit, and where schools build nap breaks into their daily schedules. Imagine a world where we no longer wear our exhaustion as a badge of honor, but instead take pride in caring for ourselves and each other.

Embracing the Nap Revolution

This is the world that the nap revolution seeks to create – a world where we recognize that rest is not a weakness, but a strength. By embracing napping as a fundamental human need, we can build a society that is healthier, happier, and more fulfilled. We can foster a culture of compassion, where we support each other in the pursuit of balance and well-being.

So let us join the nap revolution, one snooze at a time. Let us close our eyes, drift off into a blissful slumber, and awaken to a brighter, more vibrant future. The power of the nap is at our fingertips – all we must do is embrace it.

As we come to the end of this journey, let us remember that the nap is not just a momentary escape, but a gateway to a better way of living. By prioritizing rest, we open ourselves up to boundless possibilities – for our minds, our bodies, and our world. So, here's to the humble nap, and to the brighter future it promises. May we all find the courage to close our eyes, and the wisdom to open our hearts to the transformative power of rest.

Thank You for reading. Find my other enjoyable books in bookstores and online.

www.ingramcontent.com/pod-product-compliance
Lightning Source LLC
LaVergne TN
LVHW012011060526
838201LV00061B/4270